DIABETIC
Cookbook

pil

Publications International, Ltd.

Some of the products listed in this publication may be in limited distribution.

Front cover photograph and photograph on pages 7 and 60 © Shutterstock.com

Pictured on the front cover: Cauliflower Margherita Pizza *(page 61)*.

Pictured on the back cover *(counterclockwise from top left)*: Chicken Piccata *(page 88)*, Spinach Salad with Pomegranate Vinaigrette *(page 162)*, Lemon Raspberry Tiramisù *(page 184)*, and Spiced Chicken Skewers with Yogurt-Tahini Sauce *(page 24)*.

ISBN: 978-1-63938-051-0

Manufactured in China.

8 7 6 5 4 3 2 1

Microwave Cooking: Microwave ovens vary in wattage. Use the cooking times as guidelines and check for doneness before adding more time.

Let's get social!
@ @Publications_International
f @PublicationsInternational
www.pilbooks.com

Table of Contents

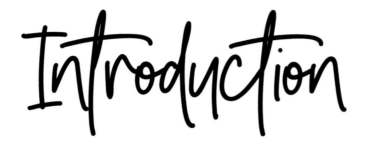

Introduction

A diagnosis of diabetes can be disheartening, but there is plenty of good news. These days, you have many diabetes tools to help you keep your blood sugar under tight control and ward off the frightening complications. You simply need to understand how to apply them to your best advantage and to commit yourself to using them faithfully.

MONITORING YOUR GLUCOSE

Blood glucose monitoring is a vital part of the diabetes management process, and frequent self-monitoring is a key to successful care. By checking your glucose, you get a precise measurement of what your blood glucose level is so you can adjust your food, medication, or activity level accordingly. Knowing your glucose level also lets you see if your previous food, medication, or activity level brought your glucose to a desired range. It means for greater freedom to participate in any activities you choose and, therefore, far greater control over your life. The blood glucose values are like clues in a mystery novel. The more clues you have, the greater your ability to solve the mystery. Of course, the opposite can be true as well. The less you check, the fewer clues you have and the more your diabetes remains a mystery to both you and your diabetes care team.

Checking your blood glucose on a regular basis allows you to know the ongoing status of your diabetes and will help you learn more about it and your body. Checking multiple times each day will give you even more information, helping you understand blood glucose patterns that occur when you eat certain foods and take specific medication doses, as well as how these are connected to your level of activity and stressors at home or work. Frequent checking also ensures that you can catch high or low levels quickly and respond to them with appropriate adjustments.

EATING FOR BETTER CONTROL

When you learned you had diabetes, you may have assumed you'd have to go on a special, restrictive diet. Perhaps you'd heard of people with diabetes who had to give up every food they enjoyed or who stopped going to certain events or restaurants because there was nothing they could eat there. Well, cheer up. You don't need to follow a "diabetic diet" anymore.

Your body needs adequate amounts of six essential nutrients to function normally. Three of these—water, vitamins, and minerals—provide no energy and do not affect blood glucose levels. The other three—carbohydrate, protein, and fat—provide your body with the energy it needs to work. This energy is measured in calories. Any food that contains calories can cause your blood glucose levels to rise. For your body to properly use these energy calories, it needs insulin. Whenever you eat, your food is digested and broken down or converted into your body's primary fuel source, glucose. While all energy nutrients are broken down into glucose, carbohydrates have a more direct effect on blood glucose levels. Protein and fat have a slower, more indirect effect on those levels. Understanding this can help you predict how food will affect your glucose levels.

To be successful in diabetes self-care, you need to make personal food choices that are compatible with your blood glucose goals and your tastes. Since carbohydrates have the greatest direct effect on glucose levels, determining the amount of carbohydrates that your body can manage well is a cornerstone in your glucose management. It's simple, really. But before you begin, you should take a close look at your perceptions, preconceptions, and habits regarding food and eating; they can make eating much more complicated than need be. Adjusting them can allow you to enjoy the freedom that simplicity brings—and allow you to enjoy eating while you control your diabetes.

To gain a better understanding of how to use food choices to control your blood sugar levels, you must pay attention to how individual foods act in your body.

The first step is for you to eat absolutely normally. Have the foods you usually eat, in the amounts you normally have, as frequently as you usually have them. Check food labels to determine which foods contain carbohydrate, then keep a running tally of the total grams of carbohydrate you eat throughout the entire day. Take detailed, honest notes.

Along with taking these notes, you need to test your blood glucose levels. Testing allows you to see how well your insulin level matches your carbohydrate intake. No matter its source, insulin works with the food you eat. If you eat too much food for the insulin that is available, your glucose level will be too high; if you eat too little, your glucose level will be too low.

It is important to know that any food has the ability to make blood sugar levels rise, but different types of food as well as different amounts will result in different blood sugar levels. You may find that overeating makes blood sugar levels increase rapidly and stay too high. Overeating may not allow insulin to do its job properly. If you listen to your body's hunger cues and respect the feeling of fullness, your blood glucose will rise more slowly and peak at a lower level. Insulin, in turn, will be able to do its job and keep blood sugars at a healthy level. This type of balanced eating helps control diabetes and helps you feel better.

Eating a variety of foods will also help ensure that you get the nutrients you need—not just the carbohydrate, protein, and fat but also the vitamins and minerals that are essential to good health.

STAYING ACTIVE

Activity is one of the three cornerstones in the treatment of diabetes, along with food and medication. Moving toward a more physically active life is generally inexpensive, convenient, and easy and usually produces great rewards in terms of blood glucose control (due to improved insulin sensitivity) and a general feeling of well-being.

Being active needs to be fun. Otherwise, you're much less likely to stick with an active lifestyle. So, choose your activities accordingly, then go out and play at least a little every day.

USING MEDICATIONS TO TREAT DIABETES

For many people who have type 2 diabetes, using food and activity to control blood glucose is not enough. For them, diabetes medications can be lifesavers—helping to lower blood glucose levels and stave off diabetes complications.

People with type 1 diabetes make very little, if any, insulin, so they are dependent on insulin injections. Insulin injections have become extremely safe and simple, and virtually pain-free. And, they remain the most natural and effective way to treat high blood sugar in these individuals.

On the other hand, individuals with type 2 diabetes may depend on pills to help lower blood glucose levels. But there are usually multiple problems that need to be addressed, and one pill just can't do it all. Problems include insulin resistance by the body's cells, oversecretion of glucose by the liver, insufficient insulin production by the pancreas, and alternated rates of food digestion. Sometimes a combination of medications is much more effective at lowering glucose levels than is a single medicine.

WEIGHING THE BENEFITS

You may realize (or your doctor has told you) that being overweight—especially carrying too much fat in your abdominal area—hampers diabetes control. For people with diabetes, the best path to weight loss is the same one that leads to getting well and staying well. There's no denying weight loss is beneficial for people with type 2 diabetes who are overweight. Even a weight loss of just 5 to 10 percent of your total body weight can bring impressive improvements to your health. Studies show that when a person who has recently been diagnosed with diabetes loses weight, blood glucose levels drop, blood pressure improves, and cholesterol levels return to a healthier range. Medications may be decreased or even stopped altogether.

TAKING COMMAND OF YOUR CARE

The right approach to diabetes treatment puts YOU in charge. Not your doctor. Not your spouse. YOU. You become the boss of your diabetes team, choosing the staff that best serves your needs, tracking your progress, and keeping your eyes on the ultimate goal— your health and well-being.

YOU'RE ON YOUR WAY

Once you feel comfortable with your meal and activity plan, checking your blood sugar, and managing your medication, you'll be able to enjoy the great taste of food without worries. Use the following recipes to get started on the path to a healthier lifestyle.

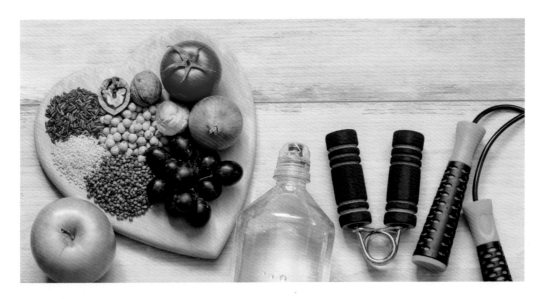

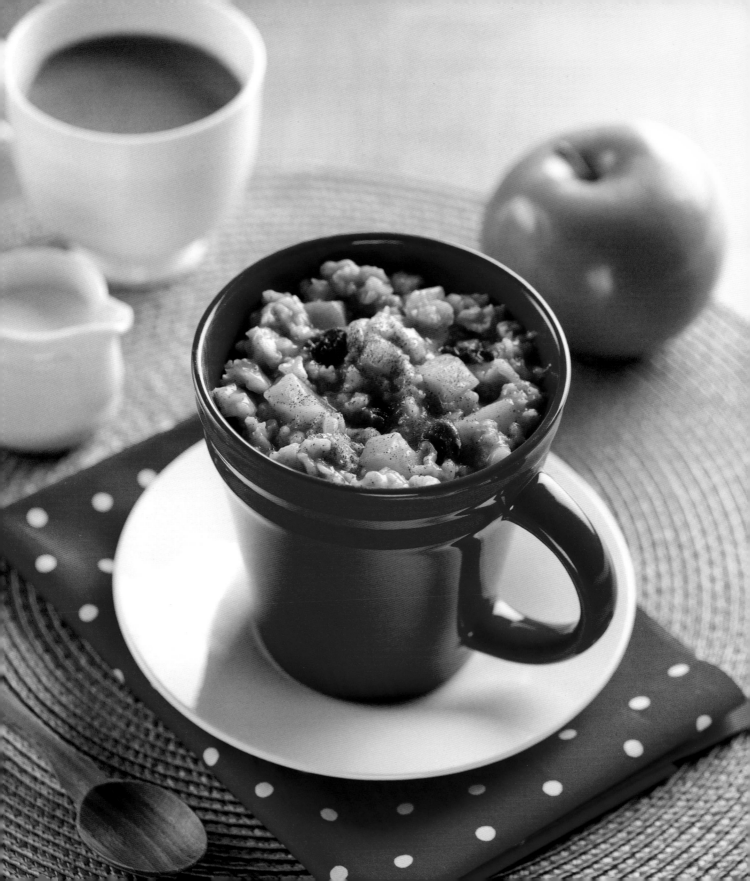

Best Breakfasts

HARVEST APPLE OATMUG
MAKES 1 SERVING

---

1 cup water

½ cup old-fashioned oats

½ cup chopped Granny Smith apple

2 tablespoons raisins

1 teaspoon packed brown sugar

¼ teaspoon ground cinnamon

⅛ teaspoon salt

MICROWAVE DIRECTIONS

1 Combine water, oats, apple, raisins, brown sugar, cinnamon and salt in large microwavable mug; mix well.

2 Microwave on HIGH 1½ minutes; stir. Microwave on HIGH 1 minute or until thickened and liquid is absorbed. Let stand 1 to 2 minutes before serving.

NUTRIENTS PER SERVING:

Calories: 251, **Total Fat:** 3g, **Saturated Fat:** 1g, **Cholesterol:** 0mg, **Sodium:** 302mg, **Carbohydrates:** 54g, **Dietary Fiber:** 6g, **Protein:** 6g
Dietary Exchange: 2 Bread/Starch, 1½ Fruit

BREAKFAST PIZZA MARGHERITA

MAKES 6 SERVINGS

---

1 (12-inch) prepared pizza crust

3 slices 95% fat-free turkey bacon

2 cups cholesterol-free egg substitute

½ cup fat-free (skim) milk

1½ tablespoons chopped fresh basil, divided

⅛ teaspoon black pepper

2 plum tomatoes, thinly sliced

½ cup (2 ounces) shredded reduced-fat mozzarella cheese

¼ cup (1 ounce) shredded reduced-fat Cheddar cheese

---

1 Preheat oven to 450°F. Place pizza crust on 12-inch pizza pan. Bake 6 to 8 minutes or until heated through.

2 Meanwhile, coat large skillet with nonstick cooking spray. Cook bacon over medium-high heat until crisp. Remove from skillet to paper towels; cool. Crumble bacon.

3 Combine egg substitute, milk, ½ tablespoon basil and pepper in medium bowl. Coat same skillet with cooking spray. Add egg substitute mixture. Cook over medium heat until mixture begins to set around edges. Gently stir eggs, allowing uncooked portions to flow underneath. Repeat stirring of egg mixture every 1 to 2 minutes or until eggs are just set. Remove from heat.

4 Arrange tomato slices on warmed pizza crust. Spoon scrambled eggs over tomatoes. Sprinkle with bacon. Top with cheese. Bake 1 minute or until cheese is melted. Sprinkle with remaining 1 tablespoon basil. Cut into 6 wedges. Serve immediately.

NUTRIENTS PER SERVING:

Calories: 311, **Total Fat:** 9g, **Saturated Fat:** 2g, **Cholesterol:** 11mg, **Sodium:** 675mg, **Carbohydrates:** 35g, **Dietary Fiber:** 2g, **Protein:** 21g
Dietary Exchange: 2 Bread/Starch, 2 Meat, ½ Vegetable, 1½ Fat

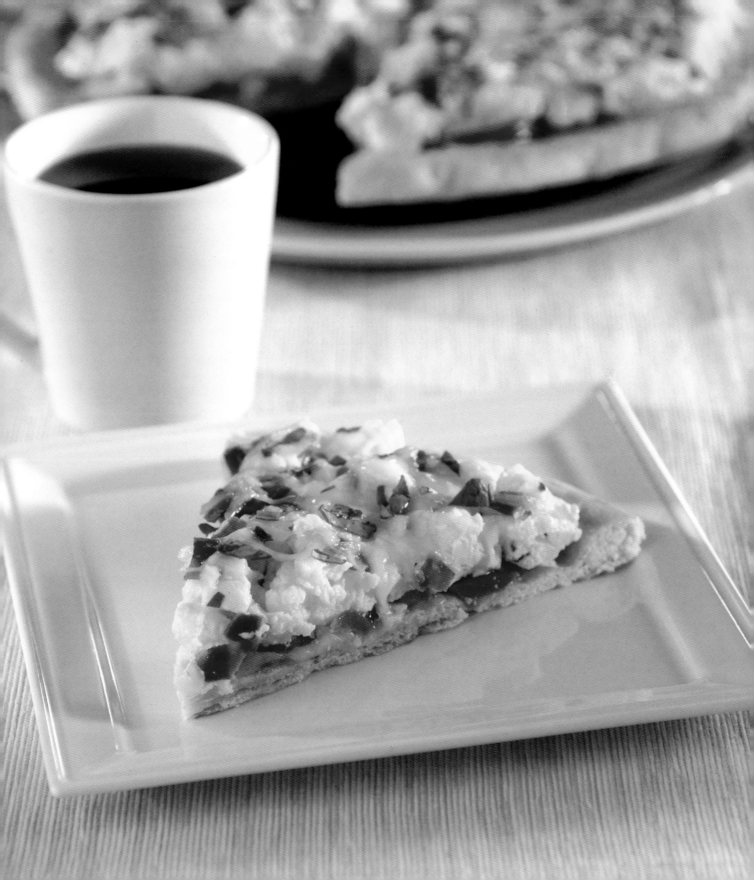

ROASTED PEPPER AND SOURDOUGH BRUNCH CASSEROLE

MAKES 8 SERVINGS

- **3** cups sourdough bread cubes
- **1** jar (12 ounces) roasted red pepper strips, drained
- **1** cup (4 ounces) shredded reduced-fat sharp Cheddar cheese
- **1** cup (4 ounces) shredded reduced-fat Monterey Jack cheese
- **1** cup fat-free cottage cheese
- **1½** cups cholesterol-free egg substitute
- **1** cup fat-free (skim) milk
- **¼** cup chopped fresh cilantro
- **¼** teaspoon black pepper

1 Lightly coat 11×7-inch baking dish with nonstick cooking spray. Place bread cubes in prepared baking dish; top with roasted peppers and shredded cheese.

2 Place cottage cheese in food processor or blender; process until smooth. Add egg substitute and milk; process just until blended. Pour over ingredients in baking dish. Sprinkle with cilantro and black pepper. Cover and refrigerate 4 hours or overnight.

3 Preheat oven to 375°F. Bake, uncovered, 40 minutes or until center is set and top is golden brown.

NUTRIENTS PER SERVING:

Calories: 179, **Total Fat:** 6g, **Saturated Fat:** 3g, **Cholesterol:** 22mg, **Sodium:** 704mg, **Carbohydrates:** 13g, **Dietary Fiber:** 1g, **Protein:** 19g
Dietary Exchange: 1 Bread/Starch, 2 Meat

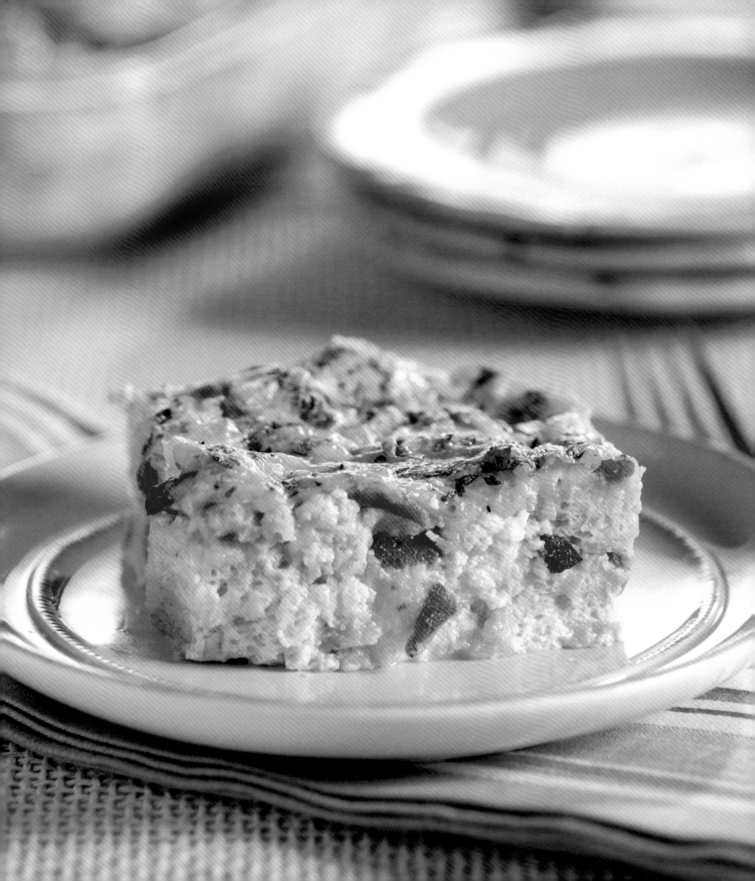

CRUSTLESS HAM & SPINACH TART

MAKES 6 SERVINGS

6 tablespoons shredded Parmesan cheese, divided

1 teaspoon olive oil

1 cup finely chopped onion

2 cloves garlic, minced

1 package (10 ounces) frozen chopped spinach, thawed and squeezed dry

3 slices deli ham, cut into strips (3 ounces total)

1¼ cups fat-free (skim) milk

¾ cup egg substitute

1½ tablespoons all-purpose flour

1 tablespoon minced fresh basil *or* 2 teaspoons dried basil

½ teaspoon black pepper

⅛ teaspoon ground nutmeg

1 Preheat oven to 350°F. Lightly spray 9-inch glass pie plate with nonstick cooking spray. Sprinkle with 2 tablespoons Parmesan cheese.

2 Heat oil in medium nonstick skillet over medium-high heat. Add onion; cook 2 minutes or until soft, stirring occasionally. Add garlic; cook 1 minute. Stir in spinach and ham, mixing well. Spread mixture evenly in prepared pie plate.

3 Combine milk, egg substitute, flour, basil, pepper and nutmeg in medium bowl; pour over spinach mixture.

4 Bake 50 minutes or until knife inserted into center comes out clean. Sprinkle with remaining 4 tablespoons Parmesan cheese.

NUTRIENTS PER SERVING:

Calories: 107, **Total Fat:** 3g, **Saturated Fat:** 1g, **Cholesterol:** 12mg, **Sodium:** 376mg, **Carbohydrates:** 9g, **Dietary Fiber:** 2g, **Protein:** 11g
Dietary Exchange: 1 Meat, 2 Vegetable

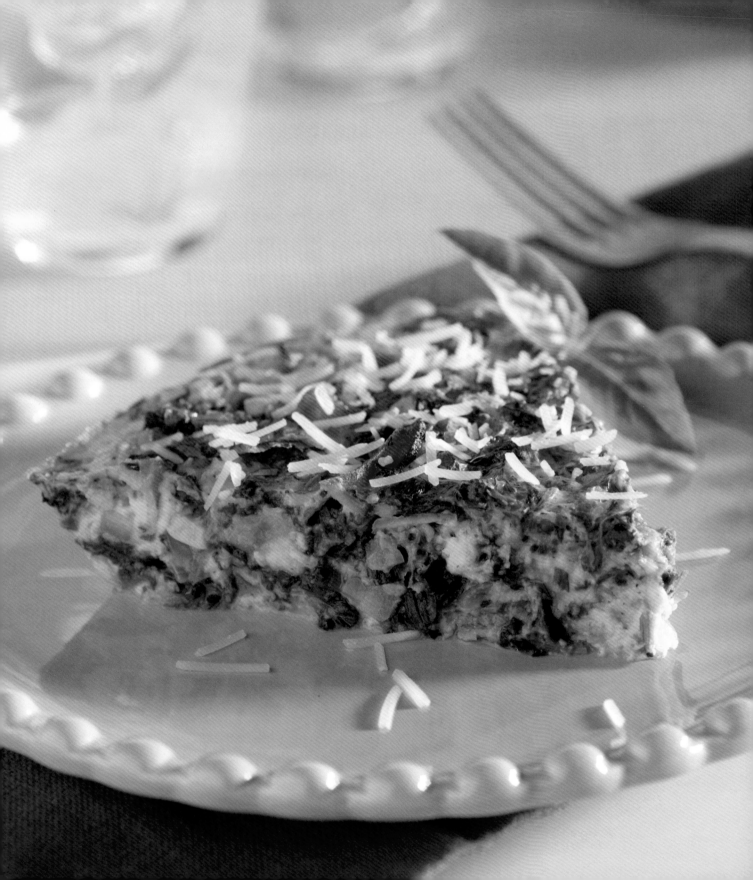

BUCKWHEAT BREAKFAST BOWL

MAKES 6 SERVINGS

3 to 4 cups reduced-fat (2%) milk*

2 tablespoons packed brown sugar

½ teaspoon vanilla

½ teaspoon ground cinnamon, divided

1 cup kasha**

2 teaspoons unsalted butter

2 apples, cut into ½-inch chunks

2 tablespoons maple syrup

¼ cup chopped walnuts

For a creamier consistency, use more milk.

**Kasha, or buckwheat groats, is buckwheat that has been pre-toasted. It is commonly found in the Kosher section of the supermarket.*

1 Combine milk, brown sugar, vanilla and ¼ teaspoon cinnamon in large saucepan. Bring to a boil over medium heat. Stir in kasha; reduce heat to low. Cook and stir 8 to 10 minutes or until kasha is tender and liquid is absorbed.

2 Meanwhile, melt butter in large nonstick skillet over medium heat. Stir in remaining ¼ teaspoon cinnamon. Add apples; cook and stir 4 to 5 minutes or until tender. Stir in maple syrup and walnuts; heat through.

3 Spoon kasha into 6 bowls. Top with apple mixture. Serve immediately.

NUTRIENTS PER SERVING:

Calories: 226, **Total Fat:** 8g, **Saturated Fat:** 3g, **Cholesterol:** 13mg, **Sodium:** 119mg, **Carbohydrates:** 34g, **Dietary Fiber:** 3g, **Protein:** 6g
Dietary Exchange: 2 Bread/Starch, 2 Fat

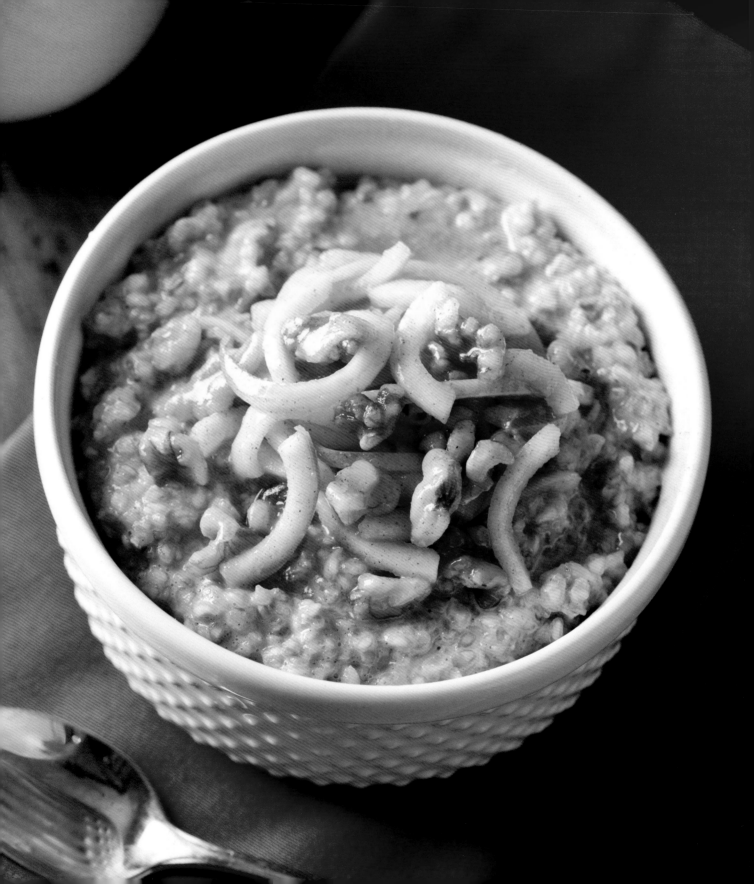

CRUSTLESS SALMON & BROCCOLI QUICHE

MAKES 4 SERVINGS

¾ cup cholesterol-free egg substitute

¼ cup chopped green onions

¼ cup plain fat-free yogurt

2 teaspoons all-purpose flour

1 teaspoon dried basil

⅛ teaspoon salt

⅛ teaspoon black pepper

¾ cup frozen broccoli florets, thawed and drained

1 can (6 ounces) boneless skinless salmon, drained and flaked

2 tablespoons grated Parmesan cheese

1 plum tomato, thinly sliced

¼ cup fresh bread crumbs

1 Preheat oven to 375°F. Spray 1½-quart casserole or 9-inch deep-dish pie plate with nonstick cooking spray.

2 Combine egg substitute, green onions, yogurt, flour, basil, salt and pepper in medium bowl until well blended. Stir in broccoli, salmon and Parmesan cheese. Spread evenly in prepared casserole. Top with tomato slices and sprinkle with bread crumbs.

3 Bake, uncovered, 20 to 25 minutes or until knife inserted near center comes out clean. Let stand 5 minutes before serving. Cut into wedges before serving.

NUTRIENTS PER SERVING:

Calories: 227, **Total Fat:** 6g, **Saturated Fat:** 2g, **Cholesterol:** 25mg, **Sodium:** 717mg, **Carbohydrates:** 20g, **Dietary Fiber:** 5g, **Protein:** 25g
Dietary Exchange: 1 Bread/Starch, 2 Meat, 1 Vegetable, ½ Fat

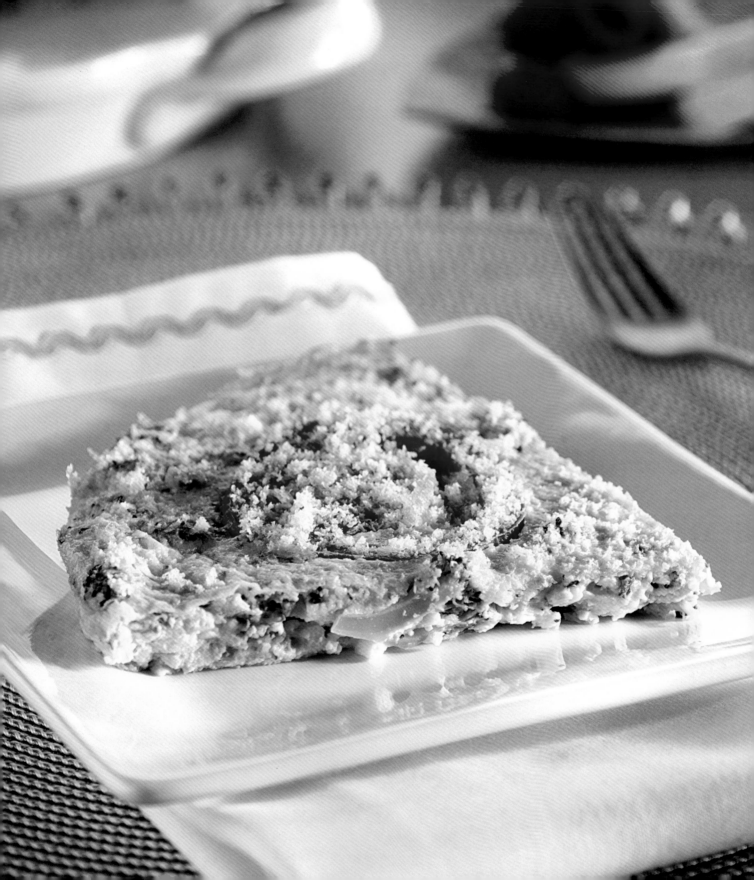

ZUCCHINI BREAD PANCAKES

MAKES 3 SERVINGS (2 PANCAKES PER SERVING)

---

1 medium zucchini, grated

¼ cup vanilla nonfat yogurt

1 egg

2 tablespoons fat-free (skim) milk

1 tablespoon vegetable oil

½ cup whole wheat flour

2 tablespoons packed brown sugar

1 teaspoon grated lemon peel, plus additional for garnish

1 teaspoon baking soda

½ teaspoon ground cinnamon

⅛ teaspoon ground nutmeg

Sugar-free maple syrup (optional)

---

1 Combine zucchini, yogurt, egg, milk and oil in large bowl; mix well. Add flour, brown sugar, 1 teaspoon lemon peel, baking soda, cinnamon and nutmeg; stir just until combined.

2 Heat large nonstick griddle or skillet over medium-low heat. Pour ¼ cupfuls of batter 2 inches apart onto griddle. Cook 3 minutes or until lightly browned and edges begin to bubble. Turn over; cook 3 minutes or until lightly browned. Repeat with remaining batter.

3 Serve with maple syrup, if desired. Garnish with additional lemon peel.

NUTRIENTS PER SERVING:

Calories: 198, **Total Fat:** 7g, **Saturated Fat:** 1g, **Cholesterol:** 63mg, **Sodium:** 468mg, **Carbohydrates:** 29g, **Dietary Fiber:** 3g, **Protein:** 7g
Dietary Exchange: 2 Bread/Starch, ½ Vegetable

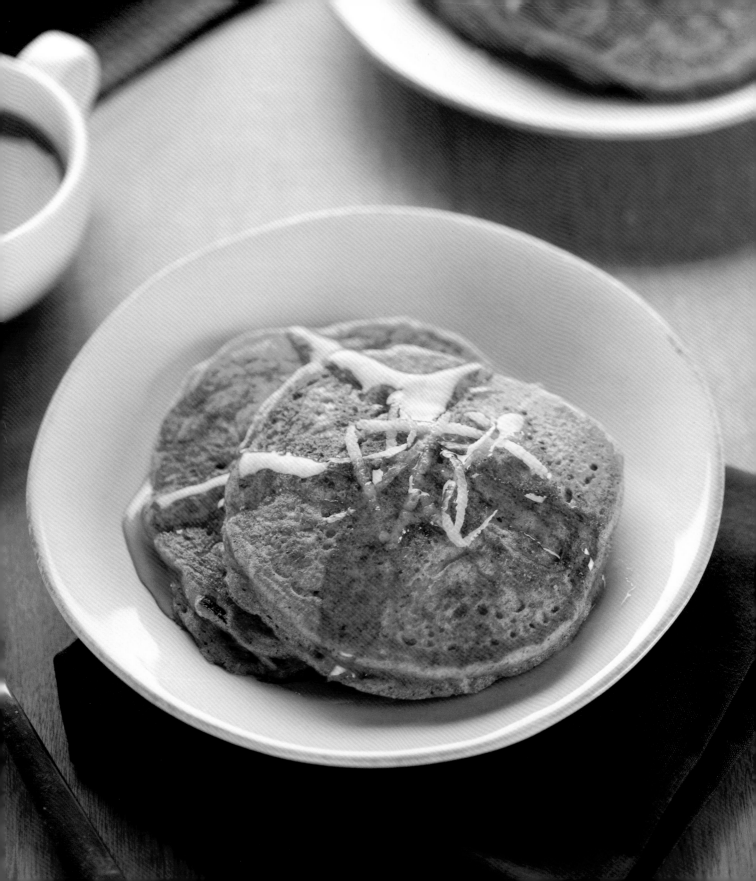

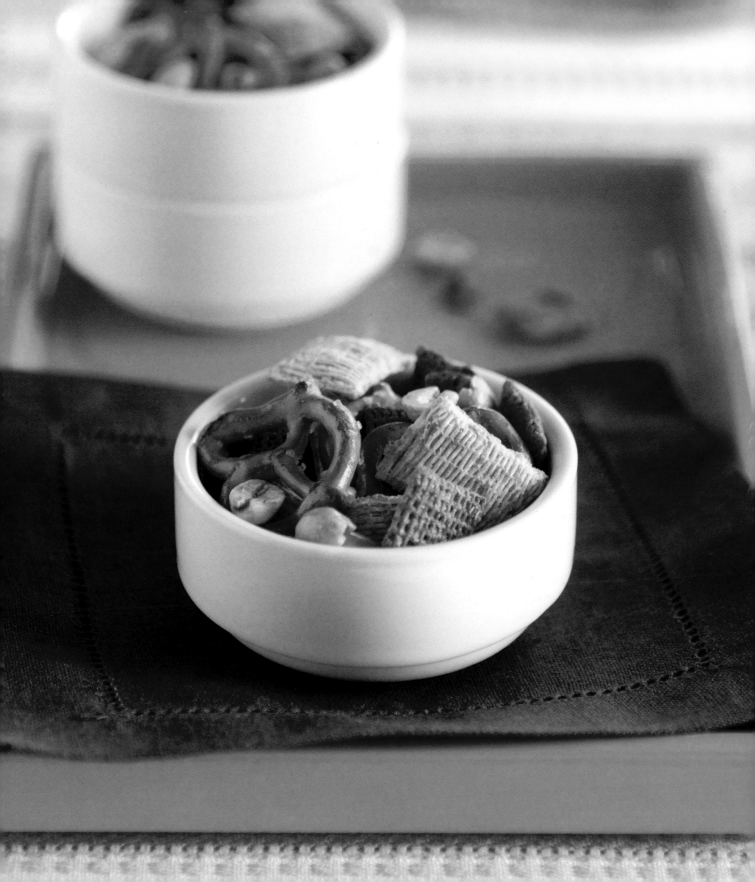

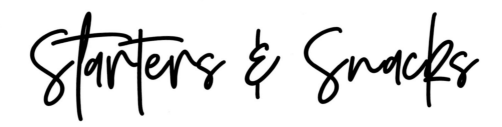
starters & snacks

SWEET & SPICY WHOLE GRAIN SNACK MIX
MAKES 10 SERVINGS

---

1 egg white

¼ cup sugar substitute*

1 tablespoon soy sauce

¼ teaspoon ground red pepper

2 cups spoon-size shredded wheat cereal

2 cups wheat cereal squares

2 cups unsalted mini-pretzel twists

¼ cup dry-roasted unsalted peanuts

This recipe was tested with sucralose-based sugar substitute.

---

1 Preheat oven to 300°F. Coat large nonstick baking pan with nonstick cooking spray; set aside.

2 Place egg white in large bowl; whisk until foamy. Whisk in sugar substitute, soy sauce and red pepper.

3 Combine cereals, pretzels and peanuts in medium bowl. Add to egg white mixture; toss to coat. Spread in even layer on prepared pan; bake 30 minutes, stirring every 10 minutes, until crispy. Cool completely on pan on wire rack. Store in airtight container for up to 1 week.

NUTRIENTS PER SERVING:

Calories: 127, **Total Fat:** 3g, **Saturated Fat:** 1g, **Cholesterol:** 0mg, **Sodium:** 216mg, **Carbohydrates:** 24g, **Dietary Fiber:** 3g, **Protein:** 4g
Dietary Exchange: 1½ Bread/Starch, ½ Fat

SPICED CHICKEN SKEWERS WITH YOGURT-TAHINI SAUCE

MAKES 8 SERVINGS

1 cup plain nonfat or regular Greek yogurt

¼ cup chopped fresh parsley, plus additional for garnish

¼ cup tahini

2 tablespoons lemon juice

1 clove garlic

¾ teaspoon salt, divided

1 tablespoon vegetable oil

2 teaspoons garam masala

1 pound boneless skinless chicken breasts, cut into 1-inch pieces

1 Prepare grill for direct cooking. Spray grid with nonstick cooking spray.

2 For sauce, combine yogurt, ¼ cup parsley, tahini, lemon juice, garlic and ¼ teaspoon salt in food processor or blender; process until smooth. Set aside.

3 Combine oil, garam masala and remaining ½ teaspoon salt in medium bowl. Add chicken; toss to coat. Thread chicken on 8 (6-inch) wooden or metal skewers.*

4 Grill chicken skewers over medium-high heat 5 minutes per side or until chicken is no longer pink. Serve with sauce. Garnish with additional parsley.

If using wooden skewers, soak in cold water 20 to 30 minutes to prevent burning.

NUTRIENTS PER SERVING:

Calories: 145, **Total Fat:** 7g, **Saturated Fat:** 1g, **Cholesterol:** 38mg, **Sodium:** 285mg, **Carbohydrates:** 4g, **Dietary Fiber:** 0g, **Protein:** 16g
Dietary Exchange: 2 Meat, 1 Fat

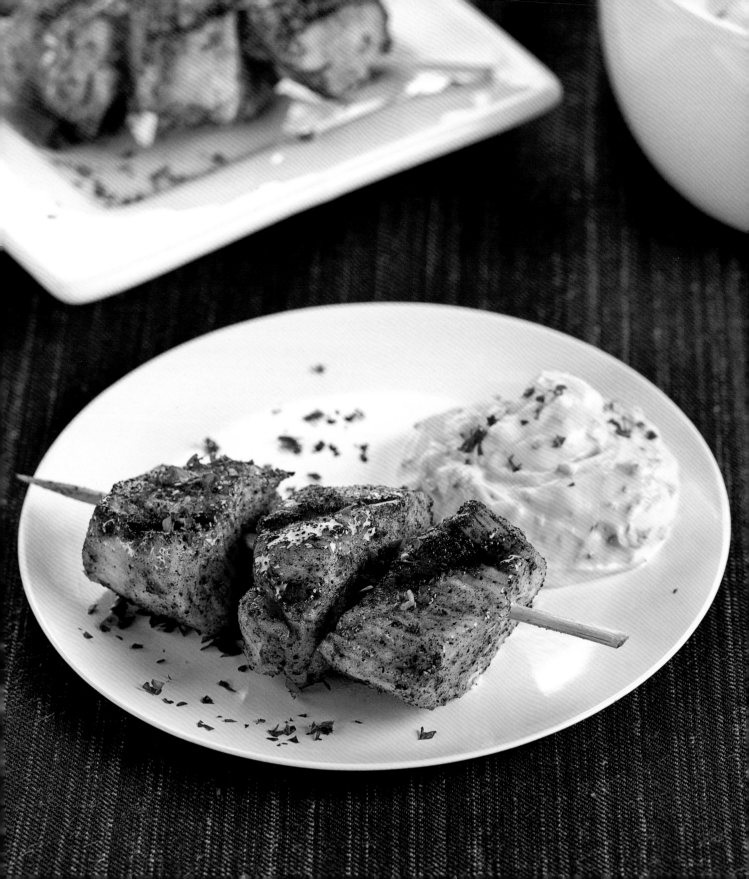

CARROT-PECAN MUFFINS

MAKES 18 MUFFINS

1 cup all-purpose flour

1 cup whole wheat flour

2 teaspoons baking powder

2 teaspoons ground cinnamon

1 teaspoon baking soda

¼ teaspoon salt

⅛ teaspoon ground cloves

2 eggs, lightly beaten

1 cup packed brown sugar

½ cup fat-free (skim) milk

¼ cup canola oil

¼ cup natural or unsweetened applesauce

1 teaspoon vanilla

2 cups finely shredded carrots

⅓ cup chopped pecans

1 Preheat oven to 375°F. Line 18 standard (2½-inch) muffin cups with paper baking cups or spray with nonstick cooking spray.

2 Combine all-purpose flour, whole wheat flour, baking powder, cinnamon, baking soda, salt and cloves in large bowl; mix well. Whisk eggs and brown sugar in medium bowl until combined. Stir in milk, oil, applesauce and vanilla until smooth. Stir into flour mixture until combined. Fold in carrots and pecans. Spoon mixture evenly into prepared muffin cups.

3 Bake 18 to 20 minutes or until toothpick inserted into centers comes out clean. Cool in pans 5 minutes. Remove to wire racks; cool completely.

NUTRIENTS PER SERVING:

Calories: 154, **Total Fat:** 5g, **Saturated Fat:** 1g, **Cholesterol:** 21mg, **Sodium:** 180mg, **Carbohydrates:** 25g, **Dietary Fiber:** 2g, **Protein:** 3g
Dietary Exchange: 1½ Bread/Starch, 1 Fat

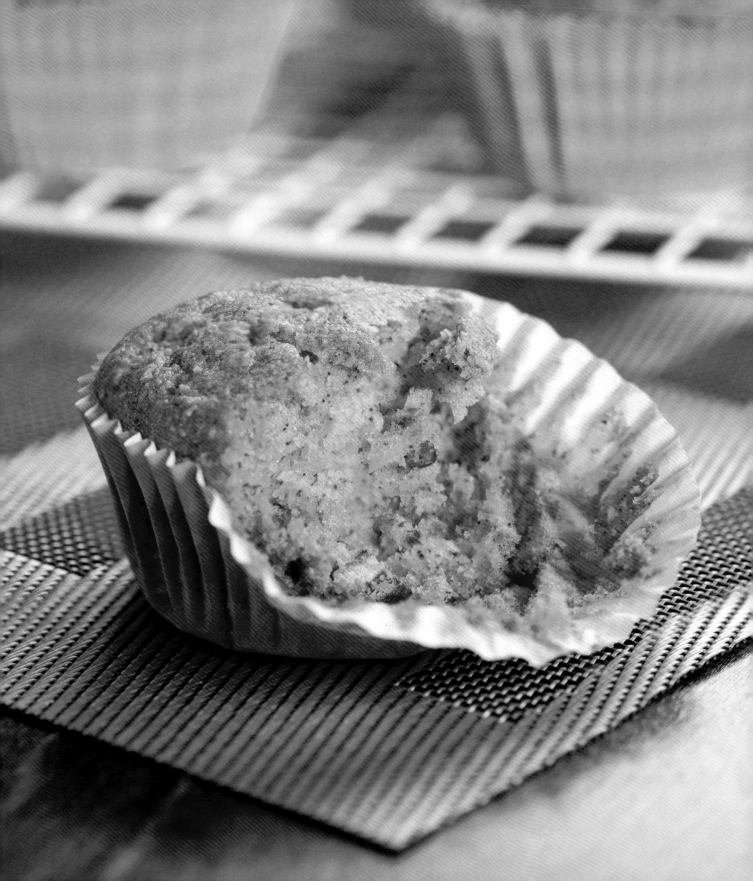

MARINATED ARTICHOKE CHEESE TOASTS

MAKES 12 SERVINGS (2 PER SERVING)

24 melba toast rounds

1 jar (8 ounces) marinated artichoke hearts, drained

½ cup (2 ounces) shredded reduced-fat Swiss cheese

⅓ cup finely chopped roasted red peppers

⅓ cup finely chopped celery

1 tablespoon plus 1½ teaspoons reduced-fat mayonnaise

Paprika (optional)

1 Preheat broiler. Place melba toast rounds on large baking sheet or broiler pan.

2 Rinse artichokes under cool running water; drain. Pat dry with paper towels.

3 Finely chop artichokes; place in medium bowl. Add cheese, peppers, celery and mayonnaise; mix well. Spoon evenly onto melba toast rounds.

4 Broil 6 inches from heat source 45 seconds or until cheese mixture is bubbly and heated through. Sprinkle with paprika, if desired.

NUTRIENTS PER SERVING:

Calories: 57, **Total Fat:** 1g, **Saturated Fat:** 1g, **Cholesterol:** 4mg, **Sodium:** 65mg, **Carbohydrates:** 7g, **Dietary Fiber:** 1g, **Protein:** 4g
Dietary Exchange: ½ Bread/Starch

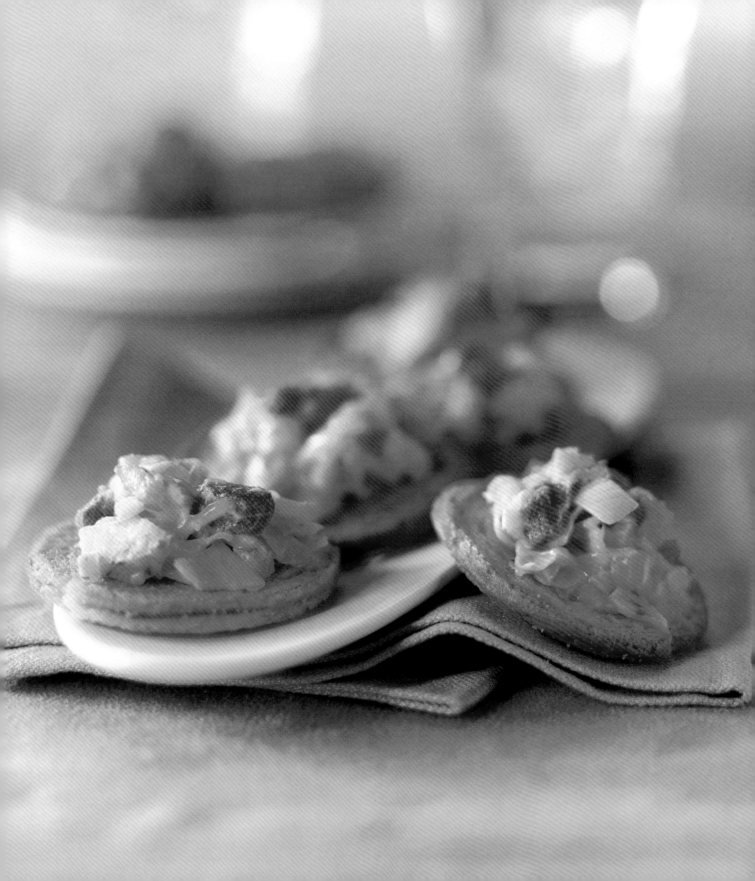

BRUSCHETTA

MAKES 4 SERVINGS

---

1 cup thinly sliced onion

½ cup chopped seeded tomato

2 tablespoons capers, drained

¼ teaspoon black pepper

3 cloves garlic, finely chopped

1 teaspoon olive oil

4 slices French bread

½ cup (2 ounces) shredded reduced-fat Monterey Jack cheese

---

1 Spray large nonstick skillet with nonstick cooking spray. Cook and stir onion over medium heat 5 minutes. Stir in tomato, capers and pepper. Cook 3 minutes.

2 Preheat broiler. Combine garlic and oil in small bowl; brush over bread slices. Top with onion mixture; sprinkle with cheese. Place on baking sheet. Broil 3 minutes or until cheese melts.

NUTRIENTS PER SERVING:

Calories: 90, **Total Fat:** 2g, **Saturated Fat:** 1g, **Cholesterol:** 0mg, **Sodium:** 194mg, **Carbohydrates:** 17g, **Dietary Fiber:** 1g, **Protein:** 3g
Dietary Exchange: 1 Bread/Starch

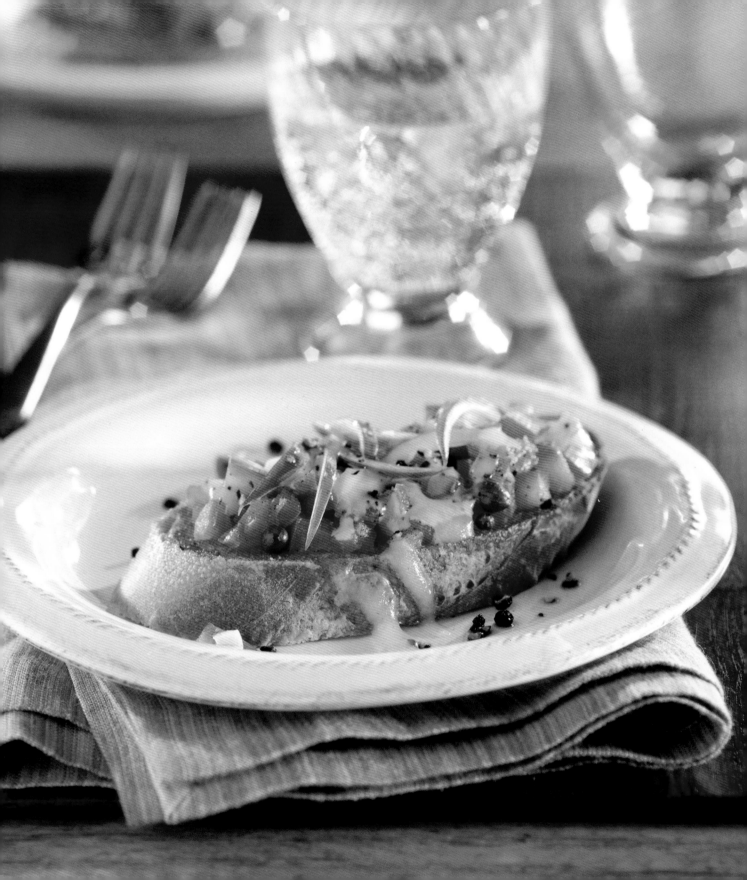

SOUTHERN CRAB CAKES WITH RÉMOULADE DIPPING SAUCE

MAKES 8 SERVINGS

---

10 ounces fresh lump crabmeat

1½ cups fresh white or sourdough bread crumbs, divided

¼ cup chopped green onions

½ cup fat-free or reduced-fat mayonnaise, divided

1 egg white, lightly beaten

2 tablespoons coarse grain or spicy brown mustard, divided

¾ teaspoon hot pepper sauce, divided

2 teaspoons olive oil, divided

Lemon wedges (optional)

---

1 Preheat oven to 200°F. Pick out and discard any shell or cartilage from crabmeat. Combine crabmeat, ¾ cup bread crumbs and green onions in medium bowl. Add ¼ cup mayonnaise, egg white, 1 tablespoon mustard and ½ teaspoon hot pepper sauce; mix well. Using ¼ cup mixture per cake, shape into 8 (½-inch-thick) cakes. Roll crab cakes lightly in remaining ¾ cup bread crumbs.

2 Heat large nonstick skillet over medium heat; add 1 teaspoon oil. Add 4 crab cakes; cook 4 to 5 minutes per side or until golden brown. Transfer to serving platter; keep warm in oven. Repeat with remaining 1 teaspoon oil and crab cakes.

3 For dipping sauce, combine remaining ¼ cup mayonnaise, 1 tablespoon mustard and ¼ teaspoon hot pepper sauce in small bowl; mix well.

4 Serve crab cakes warm with dipping sauce and lemon wedges, if desired.

NUTRIENTS PER SERVING:

Calories: 81, **Total Fat:** 2g, **Saturated Fat:** 1g, **Cholesterol:** 30mg, **Sodium:** 376mg, **Carbohydrates:** 8g, **Dietary Fiber:** 1g, **Protein:** 7g
Dietary Exchange: ½ Bread/Starch, 1 Meat

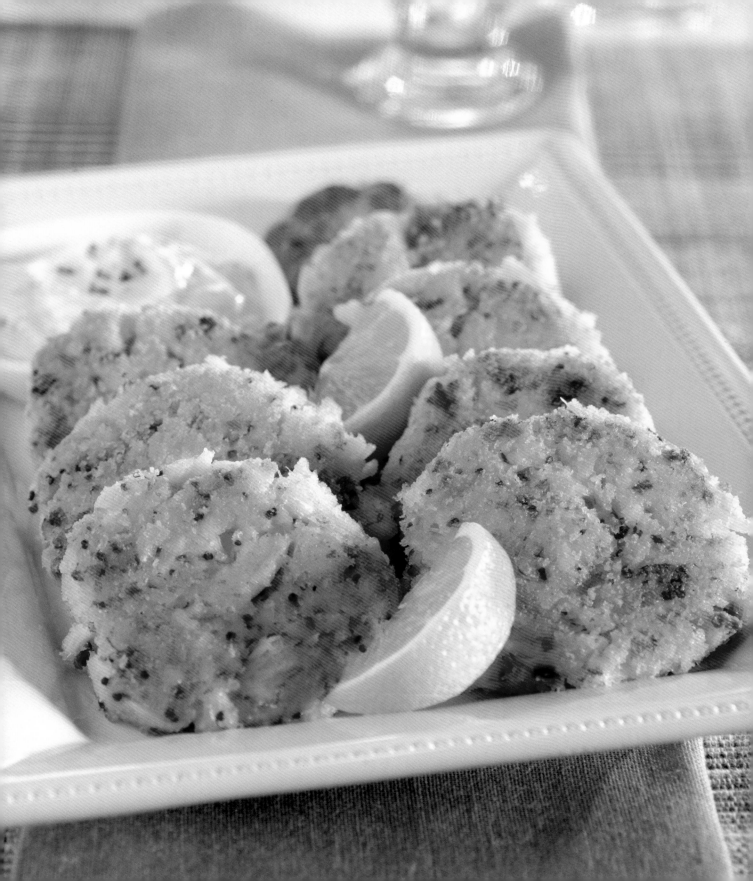

SNACKING SURPRISE MUFFINS

MAKES 12 MUFFINS

1½ cups all-purpose flour

1 cup fresh or frozen blueberries

½ cup sugar

2½ teaspoons baking powder

1 teaspoon ground cinnamon

¼ teaspoon salt

⅔ cup buttermilk

1 egg, beaten

¼ cup (½ stick) butter, melted

3 tablespoons peach preserves

TOPPING

1 tablespoon sugar

¼ teaspoon ground cinnamon

1 Preheat oven to 400°F. Line 12 standard (2½-inch) muffin pan cups with paper baking cups; set aside.

2 Combine flour, blueberries, ½ cup sugar, baking powder, 1 teaspoon cinnamon and salt in medium bowl. Combine buttermilk, egg and butter in small bowl. Add to flour mixture; mix just until moistened.

3 Spoon about 1 tablespoon batter into each muffin cup. Drop a scant teaspoonful of preserves into center of batter in each cup; top with remaining batter.

4 Combine 1 tablespoon sugar and ¼ teaspoon cinnamon in small bowl; sprinkle evenly over tops of batter.

5 Bake 18 to 20 minutes or until lightly browned. Remove muffins to wire rack to cool completely.

NUTRIENTS PER SERVING:

Calories: 156, **Total Fat:** 5g, **Saturated Fat:** 1g, **Cholesterol:** 18mg, **Sodium:** 215mg, **Carbohydrates:** 27g, **Dietary Fiber:** 1g, **Protein:** 3g
Dietary Exchange: 1½ Bread/Starch, 1 Fat

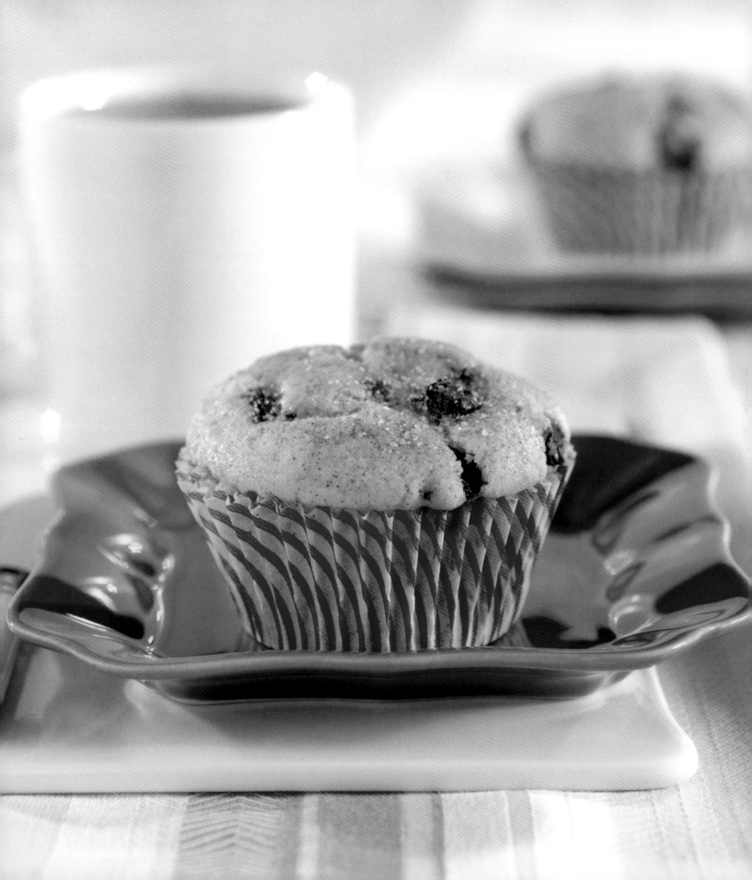

MARINATED CITRUS SHRIMP

MAKES 16 SERVINGS

1 pound (about 32) large cooked shrimp, peeled and deveined (with tails on)

2 oranges, peeled and cut into segments

1 can (5½ ounces) pineapple chunks in juice, drained and ¼ cup juice reserved

2 green onions, sliced

½ cup orange juice

2 tablespoons lime juice

2 tablespoons white wine vinegar

2 tablespoons minced fresh cilantro

1 tablespoon olive or vegetable oil

1 clove garlic, minced

½ teaspoon dried basil

½ teaspoon dried tarragon

White pepper (optional)

1 Combine shrimp, orange segments, pineapple chunks and green onions in large resealable food storage bag. Mix orange juice, reserved pineapple juice, lime juice, vinegar, cilantro, oil, garlic, basil and tarragon in medium bowl; pour over shrimp mixture, turning to coat. Season with white pepper, if desired.

2 Marinate in refrigerator 2 hours or up to 8 hours.

NUTRIENTS PER SERVING:

Calories: 51, **Total Fat:** 1g, **Saturated Fat:** 1g, **Cholesterol:** 44mg, **Sodium:** 50mg, **Carbohydrates:** 5g, **Dietary Fiber:** 1g, **Protein:** 5g
Dietary Exchange: ½ Meat, ½ Fruit

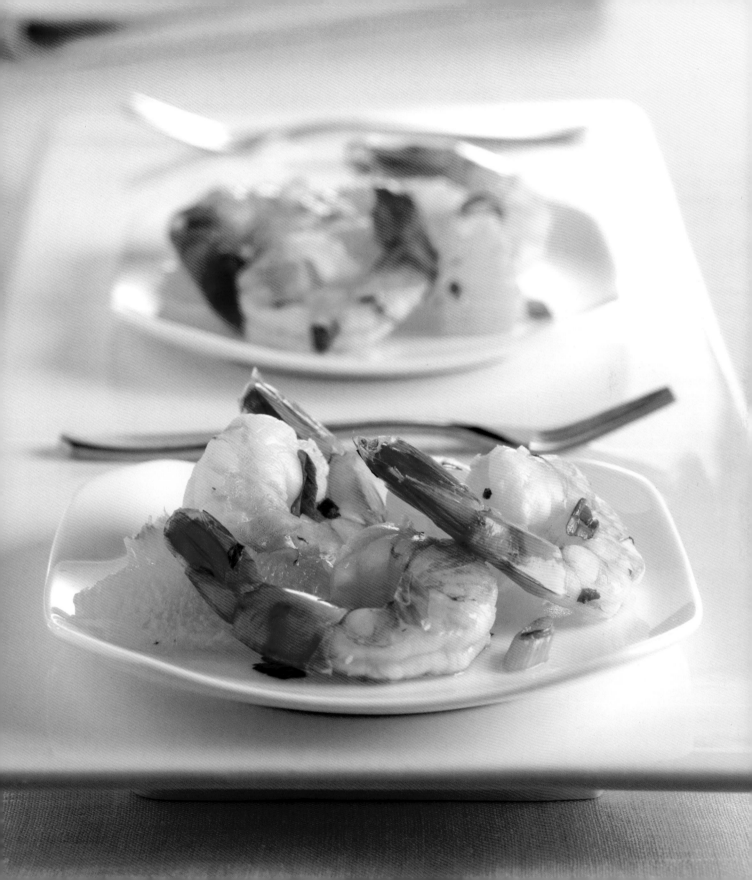

TORTELLINI TEASERS

MAKES 6 SERVINGS

Zesty Tomato Sauce (recipe follows)

½ (9-ounce) package refrigerated cheese tortellini

1 large red or green bell pepper, cut into 1-inch pieces

2 medium carrots, cut into ½-inch pieces

1 medium zucchini, cut into ½-inch pieces

12 medium mushrooms

12 cherry tomatoes

1 Prepare Zesty Tomato Sauce; keep warm.

2 Cook tortellini according to package directions. Drain.

3 Alternately thread tortellini and vegetable pieces on wooden skewers. Serve as dippers with Zesty Tomato Sauce.

ZESTY TOMATO SAUCE

MAKES ABOUT 1⅔ CUPS

1 can (15 ounces) tomato purée

2 tablespoons finely chopped onion

2 tablespoons chopped fresh parsley

1 teaspoon dried oregano

¼ teaspoon dried thyme

¼ teaspoon salt

⅛ teaspoon black pepper

Combine tomato purée, onion, parsley, oregano and thyme in small saucepan. Heat thoroughly, stirring occasionally. Stir in salt and black pepper.

NUTRIENTS PER SERVING:

Calories: 130, **Total Fat:** 2g, **Saturated Fat:** 1g, **Cholesterol:** 12mg, **Sodium:** 306mg, **Carbohydrates:** 23g, **Dietary Fiber:** 5g, **Protein:** 7g
Dietary Exchange: 1 Bread/Starch, 2 Vegetable

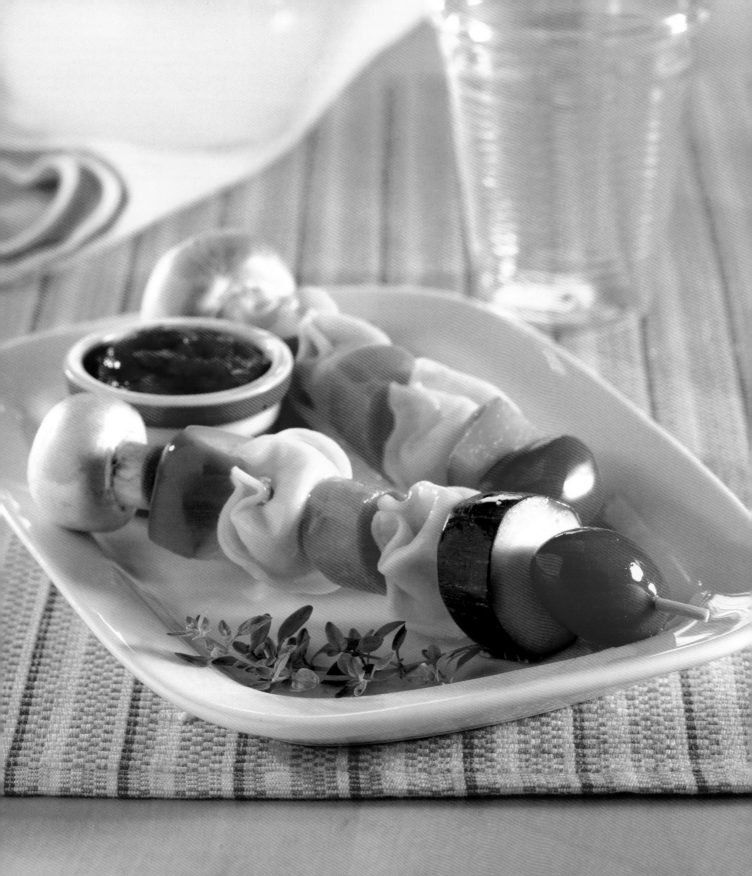

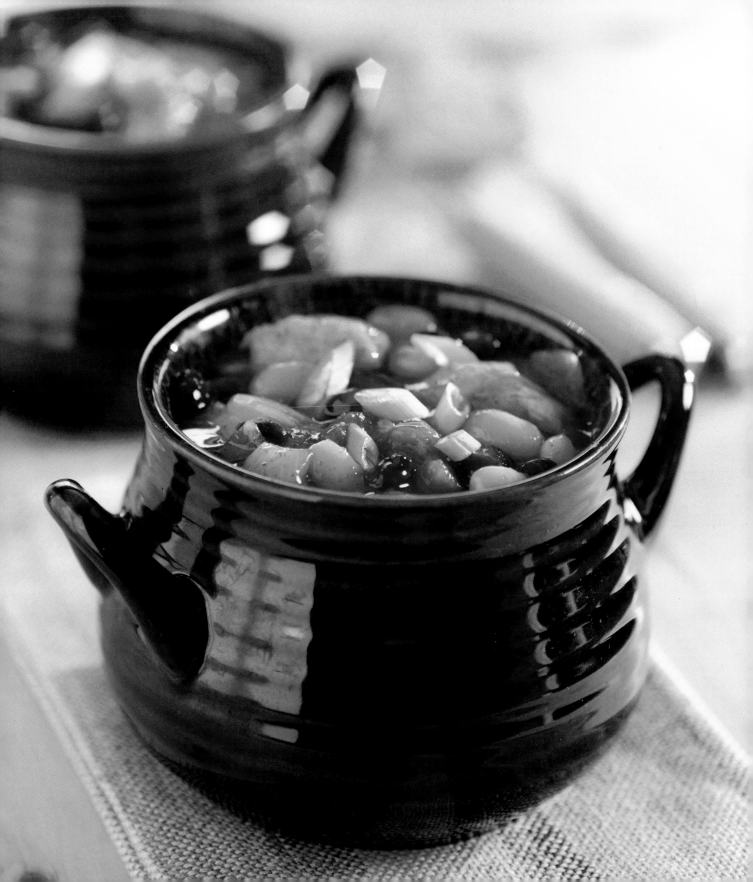

Soothing Soups

BLACK AND WHITE CHILI

MAKES 6 SERVINGS

---

1 pound chicken tenders, cut into ¾-inch pieces

1 cup coarsely chopped onion

1 can (about 15 ounces) Great Northern beans, drained

1 can (about 15 ounces) black beans, drained

1 can (about 14 ounces) Mexican-style stewed tomatoes, undrained

2 tablespoons Texas-style chili powder seasoning mix

SLOW COOKER DIRECTIONS

1 Spray large skillet with nonstick cooking spray; heat over medium heat until hot. Add chicken and onion; cook and stir 5 minutes or until chicken is browned.

2 Combine chicken mixture, beans, tomatoes with juice and chili seasoning in slow cooker. Cover; cook on LOW 4 to 4½ hours.

NUTRIENTS PER SERVING:

Calories: 260, **Total Fat:** 2g, **Saturated Fat:** 1g, **Cholesterol:** 44mg, **Sodium:** 403mg, **Carbohydrates:** 34g, **Dietary Fiber:** 8g, **Protein:** 27g
Dietary Exchange: 2 Bread/Starch, 2 Meat

SHANTUNG TWIN MUSHROOM SOUP

MAKES 6 SERVINGS

1 package (1 ounce) dried shiitake mushrooms

2 teaspoons vegetable oil

1 large onion, coarsely chopped

2 cloves garlic, minced

2 cups sliced button mushrooms

2 cans (about 14 ounces each) fat-free reduced-sodium chicken broth

2 ounces cooked ham, cut into thin slivers

½ cup thinly sliced green onions

1 tablespoon dry sherry

1 tablespoon reduced-sodium soy sauce

1 tablespoon cornstarch

1 Place shiitake mushrooms in small bowl; cover with boiling water. Let stand 20 minutes to soften. Rinse well. Drain mushrooms; squeeze out excess water. Cut off and discard stems; slice caps.

2 Heat oil in large saucepan over medium heat. Add onion and garlic. Cook and stir 1 minute. Stir in shiitake and button mushrooms; cook 4 minutes, stirring occasionally.

3 Stir in broth; bring to a boil over high heat. Reduce heat to medium; cover and simmer 15 minutes.

4 Stir in ham and green onions; cook until heated through. Stir sherry and soy sauce into cornstarch in small bowl until smooth. Add to soup; cook 2 minutes or until thickened, stirring occasionally.

NUTRIENTS PER SERVING:

Calories: 154, **Total Fat:** 4g, **Saturated Fat:** 1g, **Cholesterol:** 5mg, **Sodium:** 363mg, **Carbohydrates:** 22g, **Dietary Fiber:** 3g, **Protein:** 7g
Dietary Exchange: 1½ Bread/Starch, 1 Vegetable, ½ Fat

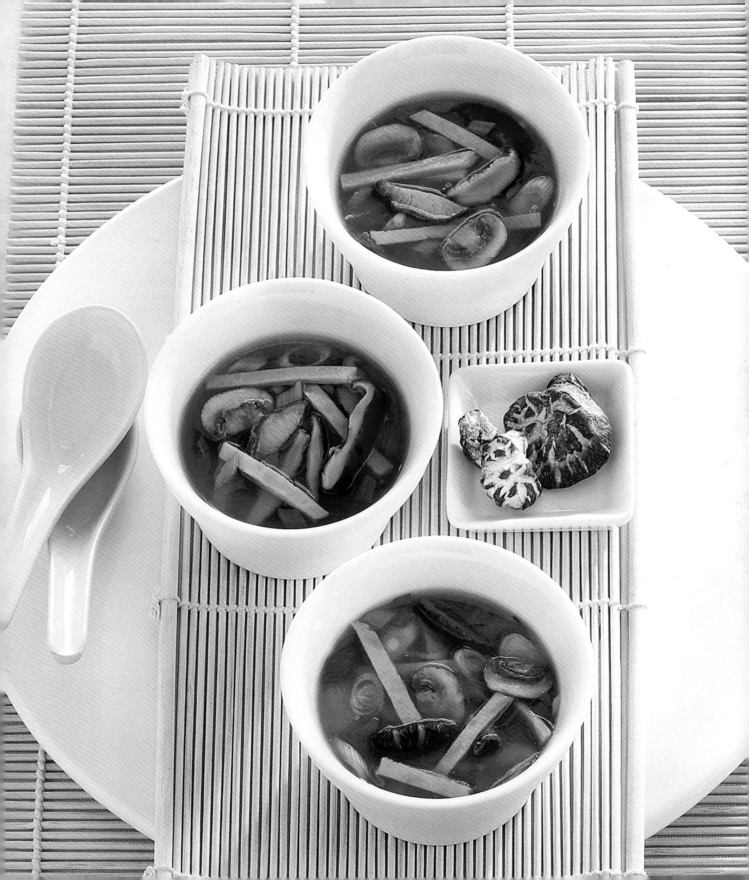

PASTA MEATBALL SOUP

MAKES 4 SERVINGS

---

10 ounces 95% lean ground beef

5 tablespoons uncooked acini di pepe pasta,* divided

¼ cup fresh fine bread crumbs

1 egg

2 tablespoons finely chopped fresh parsley, divided

1 teaspoon dried basil, divided

1 clove garlic, minced

¼ teaspoon salt

⅛ teaspoon black pepper

2 cans (about 14 ounces each) fat-free reduced-sodium beef broth

1 can (about 8 ounces) tomato sauce

⅓ cup chopped onion

Acini di pepe is tiny rice-shaped pasta. Orzo or pastina can be substituted.

---

1 Combine beef, 2 tablespoons pasta, bread crumbs, egg, 1 tablespoon parsley, ½ teaspoon basil, garlic, salt and pepper in medium bowl. Shape into 28 to 30 (1-inch) meatballs.

2 Bring broth, tomato sauce, onion and remaining ½ teaspoon basil to a boil in large saucepan over medium-high heat. Carefully add meatballs to broth mixture. Reduce heat to medium-low; simmer, covered, 20 minutes.

3 Add remaining 3 tablespoons pasta; cook 10 minutes or until tender. Garnish with remaining 1 tablespoon parsley.

NUTRIENTS PER SERVING:

Calories: 216, **Total Fat:** 7g, **Saturated Fat:** 2g, **Cholesterol:** 89mg, **Sodium:** 599mg, **Carbohydrates:** 15g, **Dietary Fiber:** 1g, **Protein:** 22g
Dietary Exchange: 1 Bread/Starch, 2½ Meat

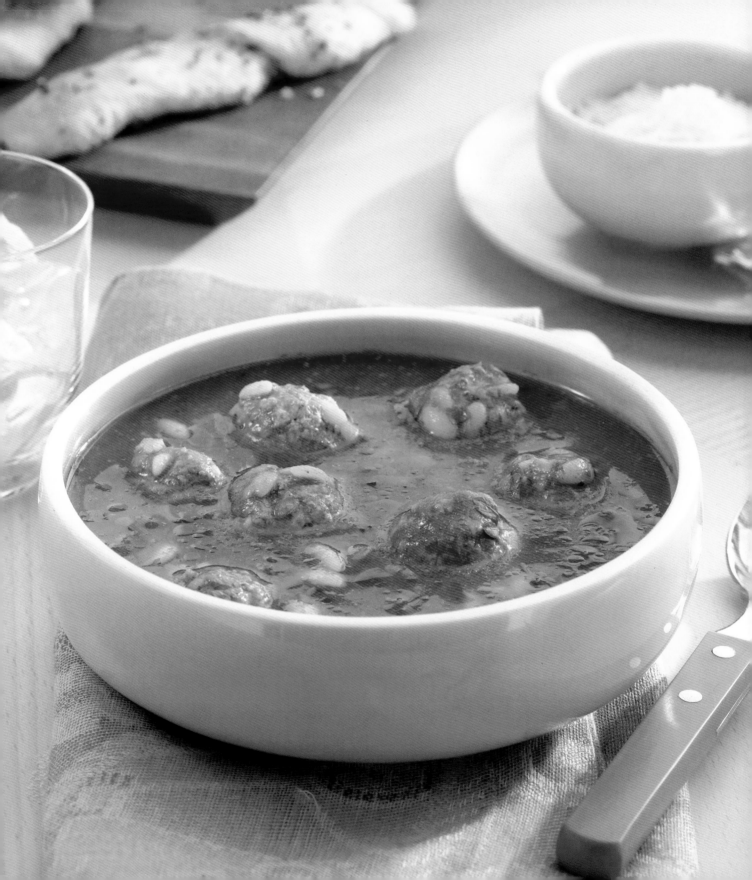

QUICK BROCCOLI SOUP

MAKES 6 SERVINGS

---

4 cups fat-free reduced-sodium chicken or vegetable broth

2½ pounds broccoli florets

1 onion, quartered

1 cup low-fat (1%) milk

¼ teaspoon salt (optional)

¼ cup crumbled blue cheese

---

1 Place broth, broccoli and onion in large saucepan; bring to a boil over high heat. Reduce heat to low; cover and simmer 20 minutes or until vegetables are tender.

2 Blend soup with hand-held immersion blender until smooth. (Or process soup in batches in food processor or blender.) Stir in milk and salt, if desired. Add water or additional broth, if needed.

3 Ladle soup into serving bowls; sprinkle with cheese.

NUTRIENTS PER SERVING:

Calories: 91, **Total Fat:** 2g, **Saturated Fat:** 1g, **Cholesterol:** 6mg, **Sodium:** 175mg, **Carbohydrates:** 12g, **Dietary Fiber:** 3g, **Protein:** 7g
Dietary Exchange: 1 Meat, 2 Vegetable

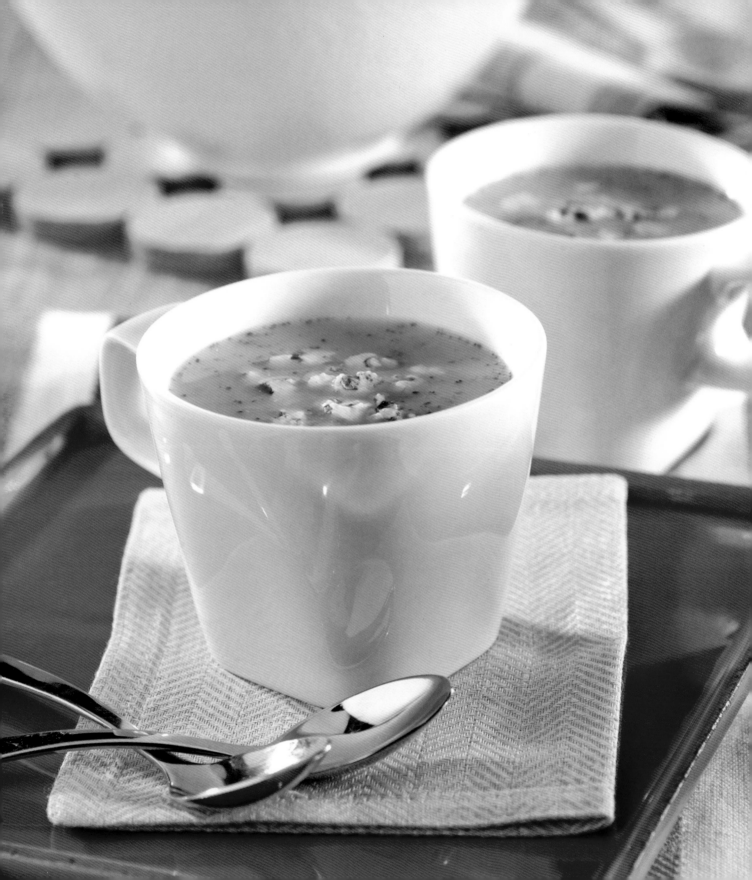

WHITE BEAN AND ESCAROLE SOUP

MAKES 6 SERVINGS

1½ cups dried baby lima beans, rinsed and sorted

1 teaspoon olive oil

½ cup chopped celery

⅓ cup coarsely chopped onion

2 cloves garlic, minced

2 cans (about 14 ounces each) no-salt-added whole tomatoes, undrained and chopped

½ cup chopped fresh parsley

2 tablespoons chopped fresh rosemary

¼ teaspoon black pepper

3 cups shredded fresh escarole

1. Place dried lima beans in large glass bowl; cover completely with water. Soak 6 to 8 hours or overnight. Drain beans; place in large saucepan or Dutch oven. Cover beans with about 3 cups water; bring to a boil over high heat. Reduce heat to low. Cover and simmer about 1 hour or until soft. Drain; set aside.

2. Heat oil in small skillet over medium heat. Add celery, onion and garlic; cook and stir 5 minutes or until onion is tender. Remove from heat.

3. Add celery mixture and tomatoes with juice to beans. Stir in parsley, rosemary and pepper. Simmer, covered, over low heat 15 minutes. Add escarole; simmer 5 minutes.

TIP: Store dried lima beans (also known as butter beans) in an airtight container in a cool, dry place for up to 1 year. When soaking, do not allow beans to soak for longer than 12 hours or they may start to ferment.

NUTRIENTS PER SERVING:

Calories: 196, **Total Fat:** 2g, **Saturated Fat:** 0g, **Cholesterol:** 0mg, **Sodium:** 33mg, **Carbohydrates:** 35g, **Dietary Fiber:** 5g, **Protein:** 12g
Dietary Exchange: 2 Bread/Starch, 2 Vegetable

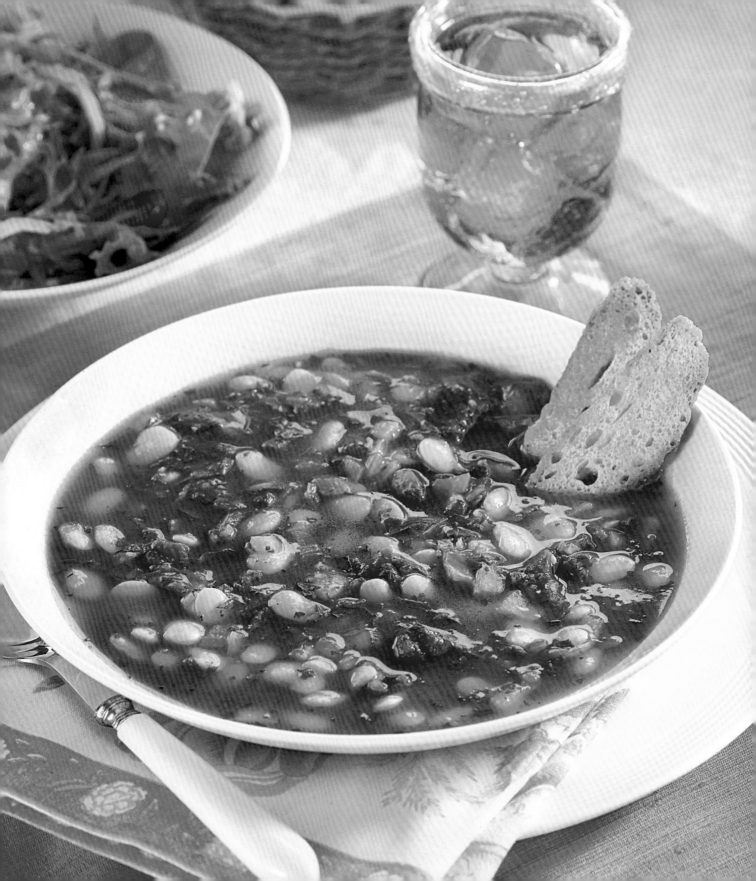

SLOW COOKER VEGGIE STEW

MAKES 4 SERVINGS

1 tablespoon vegetable oil

⅔ cup carrot slices

½ cup diced onion

2 cloves garlic, chopped

2 cans (about 14 ounces each) vegetable broth

1½ cups chopped green cabbage

½ cup cut green beans

½ cup diced zucchini

1 tablespoon tomato paste

½ teaspoon dried basil

½ teaspoon dried oregano

¼ teaspoon salt

SLOW COOKER DIRECTIONS

1 Heat oil in medium skillet over medium-high heat. Add carrots, onion and garlic; cook and stir until tender. Transfer to slow cooker.

2 Stir in remaining ingredients. Cover; cook on LOW 8 to 10 hours or on HIGH 4 to 5 hours.

NUTRIENTS PER SERVING:

Calories: 80, **Total Fat:** 3.5g, **Saturated Fat:** 0.5g, **Cholesterol:** 0mg, **Sodium:** 370mg, **Carbohydrates:** 11g, **Dietary Fiber:** 3g, **Protein:** 2g
Dietary Exchange: 2 Vegetable, 1 Fat

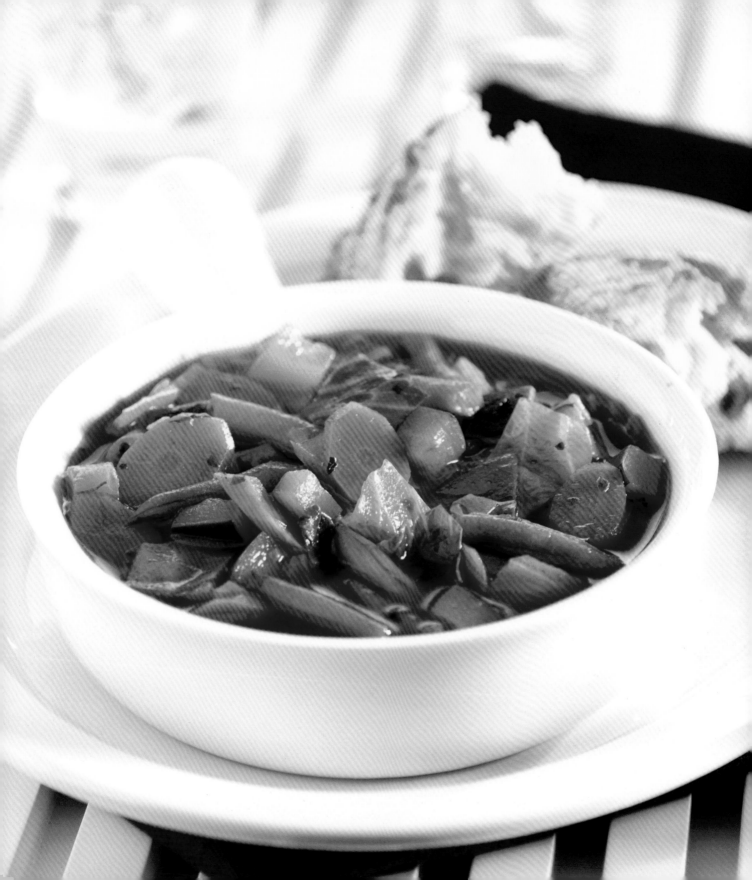

GROUND BEEF, SPINACH AND BARLEY SOUP

MAKES 4 SERVINGS

---

12 ounces 95% lean ground beef

4 cups water

1 can (about 14 ounces) stewed tomatoes

1½ cups thinly sliced carrots

1 cup chopped onion

½ cup uncooked quick-cooking barley

1½ teaspoons beef bouillon granules

1½ teaspoons dried thyme

1 teaspoon dried oregano

½ teaspoon garlic powder

¼ teaspoon black pepper

⅛ teaspoon salt

3 cups fresh spinach leaves

---

1 Brown beef in large saucepan over medium-high heat 6 to 8 minutes, stirring to break up meat. Rinse beef under warm water; drain.

2 Return beef to saucepan; stir in 4 cups water, tomatoes, carrots, onion, barley, bouillon, thyme, oregano, garlic powder, pepper and salt; bring to a boil over high heat.

3 Reduce heat to medium-low. Cover; simmer 12 to 15 minutes or until barley and vegetables are tender, stirring occasionally. Stir in spinach; cook until spinach starts to wilt.

NUTRIENTS PER SERVING:

Calories: 290, Total Fat: 5g, Saturated Fat: 2g, Cholesterol: 55mg, Sodium: 790mg, Carbohydrates: 39g, Dietary Fiber: 9g, Protein: 24g
Dietary Exchange: 1 Bread/Starch, 2 Meat

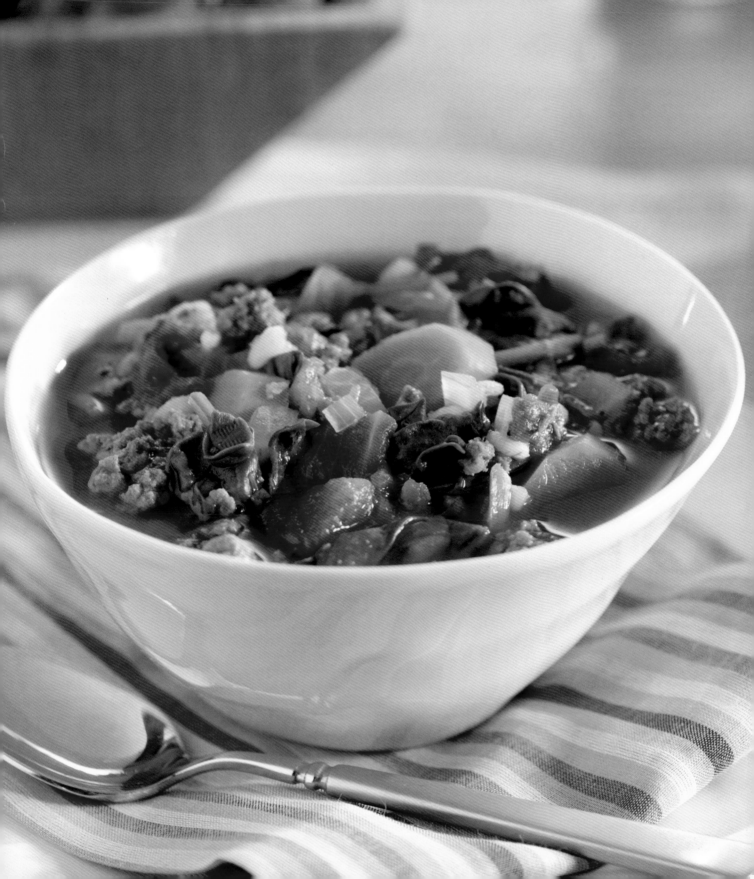

ITALIAN FISH SOUP

MAKES 2 SERVINGS

---

1 cup meatless pasta sauce

¾ cup water

¾ cup fat-free reduced-sodium chicken broth

1 teaspoon Italian seasoning

¾ cup uncooked small pasta shells

4 ounces fresh halibut or haddock steak, 1 inch thick, skinned and cut into 1-inch pieces

1½ cups frozen vegetable blend, such as broccoli, carrots and water chestnuts or broccoli, carrots and cauliflower

---

1 Combine pasta sauce, water, broth and Italian seasoning in medium saucepan; bring to a boil over high heat. Stir in pasta; return to a boil. Reduce heat to medium-low; cover and simmer 5 minutes.

2 Stir in fish and frozen vegetables; return to a boil. Reduce heat to medium-low; cover and simmer 4 to 5 minutes or until pasta is tender and fish begins to flake when tested with fork.

NUTRIENTS PER SERVING:

Calories: 331, **Total Fat:** 8g, **Saturated Fat:** 1g, **Cholesterol:** 1mg, **Sodium:** 734mg, **Carbohydrates:** 44g, **Dietary Fiber:** 4g, **Protein:** 21g
Dietary Exchange: 2 Bread/Starch, 2 Meat, 3 Vegetable

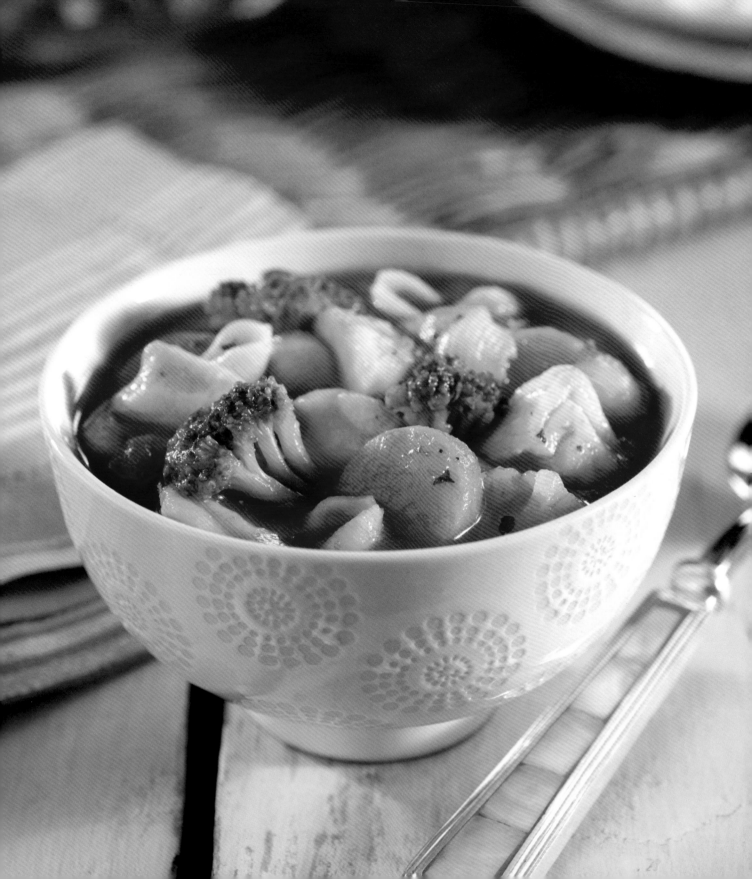

FRESH TOMATO PASTA SOUP

MAKES 8 SERVINGS

1 tablespoon olive oil

½ cup chopped onion

1 clove garlic, minced

3 pounds fresh tomatoes (about 9 medium), coarsely chopped

3 cups fat-free reduced-sodium chicken broth

1 tablespoon minced fresh basil

1 tablespoon minced fresh marjoram

1 tablespoon minced fresh oregano

1 teaspoon whole fennel seeds

½ teaspoon black pepper

¾ cup uncooked rosamarina, orzo or other small pasta

½ cup (2 ounces) shredded part-skim mozzarella cheese

1 Heat oil in large saucepan over medium heat. Add onion and garlic; cook and stir until onion is tender.

2 Add tomatoes, broth, basil, marjoram, oregano, fennel seeds and pepper; bring to a boil. Reduce heat to low; cover and simmer 25 minutes. Remove from heat; cool slightly.

3 Purée tomato mixture in batches in food processor or blender. Return to saucepan; bring to a boil. Add pasta; cook 7 to 9 minutes or until tender. Sprinkle with cheese.

NUTRIENTS PER SERVING:

Calories: 116, **Total Fat:** 4g, **Saturated Fat:** 1g, **Cholesterol:** 4mg, **Sodium:** 62mg, **Carbohydrates:** 17g, **Dietary Fiber:** 2g, **Protein:** 5g
Dietary Exchange: ½ Bread/Starch, 2 Vegetable, ½ Fat

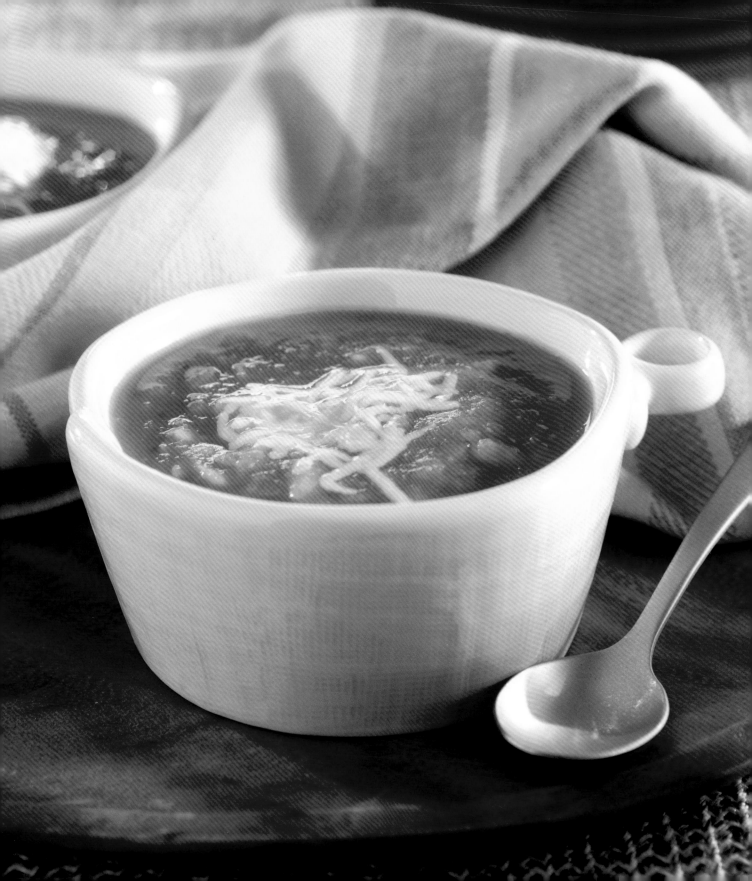

CHICKPEA-VEGETABLE SOUP

MAKES 4 SERVINGS

- 1 teaspoon olive oil
- 1 cup chopped onion
- ½ cup chopped green bell pepper
- 2 cloves garlic, minced
- 2 cans (about 14 ounces each) no-salt-added chopped tomatoes
- 3 cups water
- 2 cups broccoli florets
- 1 can (about 15 ounces) chickpeas, rinsed, drained and slightly mashed
- ½ cup (3 ounces) uncooked orzo or rosamarina pasta
- 1 bay leaf
- 1 tablespoon chopped fresh thyme *or* 1 teaspoon dried thyme
- 1 tablespoon chopped fresh rosemary *or* 1 teaspoon dried rosemary
- 1 tablespoon lime or lemon juice
- ½ teaspoon ground turmeric
- ¼ teaspoon salt
- ¼ teaspoon ground red pepper
- ¼ cup pepitas (pumpkin seeds) or sunflower kernels

---

1 Heat oil in large saucepan over medium heat. Add onion, bell pepper and garlic; cook and stir 5 minutes or until vegetables are tender.

2 Add tomatoes, water, broccoli, chickpeas, orzo, bay leaf, thyme, rosemary, lime juice, turmeric, salt and ground red pepper. Bring to a boil over high heat. Reduce heat to medium-low; cover and simmer 10 to 12 minutes or until orzo is tender.

3 Remove and discard bay leaf. Ladle soup into 4 serving bowls; sprinkle with pepitas.

NUTRIENTS PER SERVING:

Calories: 300, **Total Fat:** 6g, **Saturated Fat:** 1g, **Cholesterol:** 0mg, **Sodium:** 280mg, **Carbohydrates:** 48g, **Dietary Fiber:** 9g, **Protein:** 13g
Dietary Exchange: 2 Bread/Starch, 3 Vegetable, 1 Fat

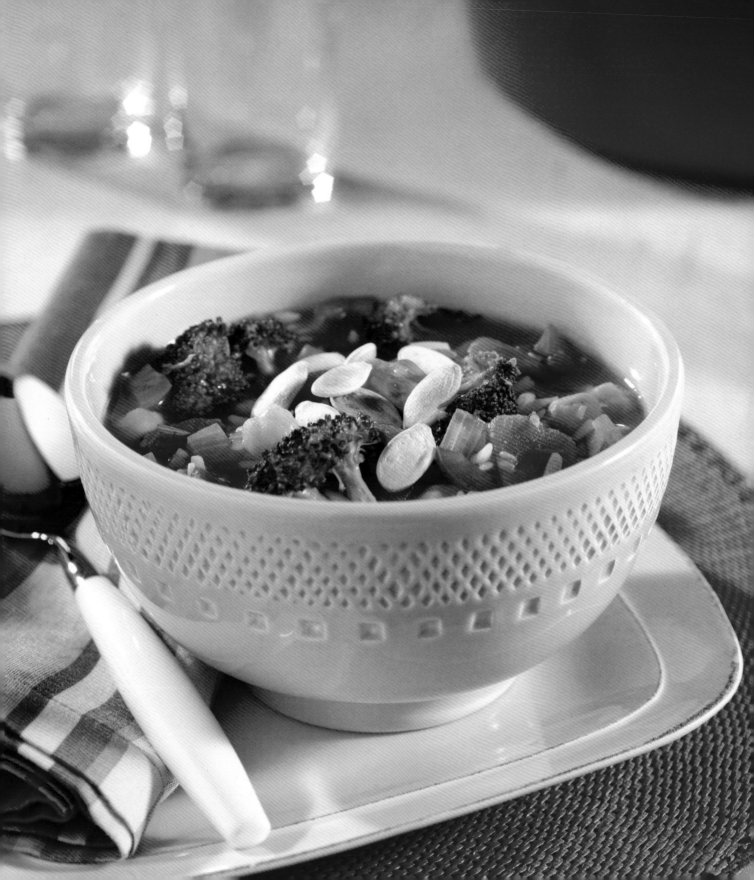

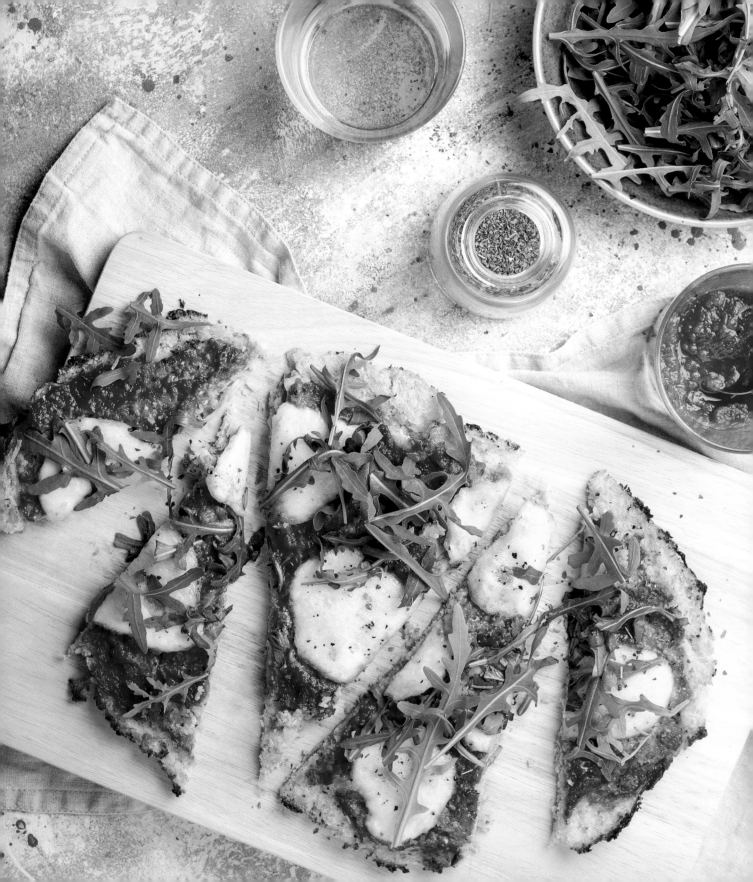

Light Bites & Midday Meals

CAULIFLOWER MARGHERITA PIZZA
MAKES 6 SERVINGS

2½ **cups finely chopped fresh cauliflower (about ½ head)***

1 **cup (4 ounces) shredded part-skim mozzarella cheese**

1 **egg**

4 **teaspoons chopped fresh oregano, divided**

2 **teaspoons olive oil**

3 **tablespoons pasta sauce, any flavor**

8 **ounces fresh part-skim mozzarella cheese, sliced**

1 **package (5 ounces) baby arugula**

Dash red pepper flakes

*To chop cauliflower easily, place in food processor and pulse until finely chopped.

---

1 Preheat oven to 450°F. Spray pizza pan with nonstick cooking spray. Line large baking sheet with foil.

2 Place cauliflower in medium microwavable bowl; microwave on HIGH 4 minutes. Stir; microwave on HIGH 4 minutes or until tender. Let cool slightly.

3 Add shredded cheese, egg and 2 teaspoons oregano to cauliflower; mix well. Pat mixture into 9-inch circle in prepared pizza pan; spray with cooking spray.

4 Bake crust 10 to 12 minutes or until golden brown around edges.

5 Spread pasta sauce over crust; top with slices of mozzarella cheese. Bake 6 to 7 minutes or until cheese is melted. Sprinkle with arugula and red pepper flakes, if desired. Cut into 6 wedges.

NUTRIENTS PER SERVING:

Calories: 220, **Total Fat:** 14g, **Saturated Fat:** 18g, **Cholesterol:** 75mg, **Sodium:** 370mg, **Carbohydrates:** 5g, **Dietary Fiber:** 1g, **Protein:** 17g
Dietary Exchange: 2½ Meat, ½ Vegetable, 2 Fat

SALMON PASTA SALAD

MAKES 2 SERVINGS

1 cup cooked medium pasta shells

1 can (about 6 ounces) canned red salmon, drained

½ cup finely chopped celery

2 tablespoons finely chopped red bell pepper

2 tablespoons chopped fresh parsley

2 tablespoons fat-free mayonnaise

1 green onion, finely chopped

1 tablespoon lemon juice

2 teaspoons capers

⅛ teaspoon paprika

Combine all ingredients in medium bowl. Cover; refrigerate until ready to serve.

NUTRIENTS PER SERVING:

Calories: 262, **Total Fat:** 9g, **Saturated Fat:** 2g, **Cholesterol:** 21mg, **Sodium:** 627mg, **Carbohydrates:** 26g, **Dietary Fiber:** 2g, **Protein:** 18g
Dietary Exchange: 1½ Bread/Starch, 2 Meat, 1 Vegetable, ½ Fat

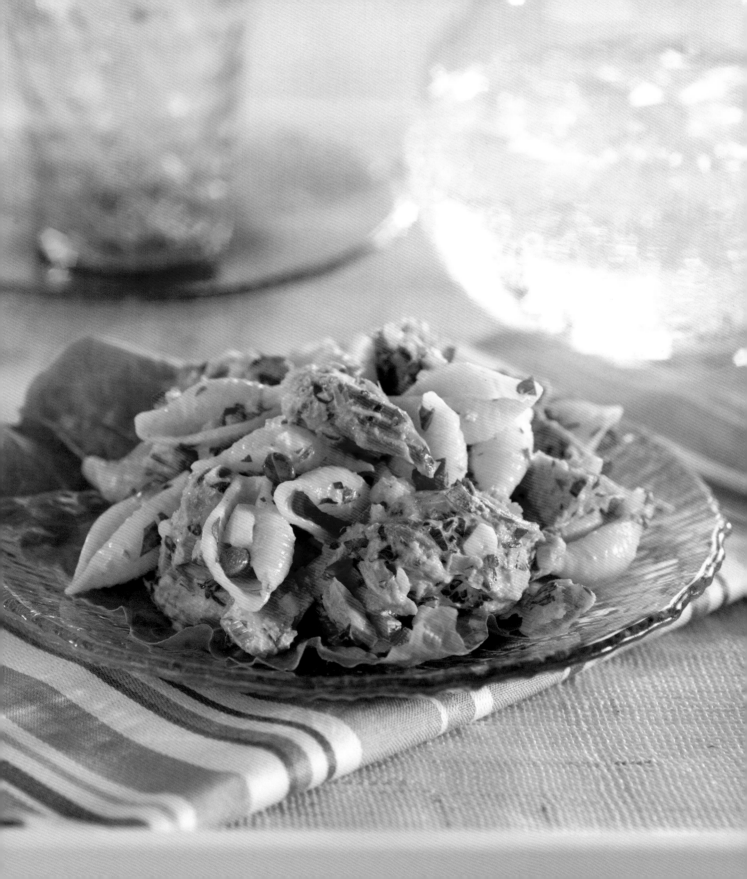

LENTIL BURGERS

MAKES 4 SERVINGS

1 can (about 14 ounces) vegetable broth

1 cup dried lentils, rinsed and sorted

1 small carrot, grated

¼ cup coarsely chopped mushrooms

1 egg

¼ cup plain dry bread crumbs

3 tablespoons finely chopped onion

2 to 4 cloves garlic, minced

1 teaspoon dried thyme

¼ cup plain fat-free yogurt

¼ cup chopped seeded cucumber

½ teaspoon dried mint

¼ teaspoon dried dill weed

¼ teaspoon black pepper

⅛ teaspoon salt

Dash hot pepper sauce (optional)

Kaiser rolls (optional)

1 Bring broth to a boil in medium saucepan over high heat. Stir in lentils; reduce heat to low. Simmer, covered, about 30 minutes or until lentils are tender and liquid is absorbed. Cool to room temperature.

2 Place lentils, carrot and mushrooms in food processor or blender; process until finely chopped but not smooth. (Some whole lentils should still be visible.) Stir in egg, bread crumbs, onion, garlic and thyme. Refrigerate, covered, 2 to 3 hours.

3 Shape lentil mixture into 4 (½-inch-thick) patties. Spray large skillet with nonstick cooking spray; heat over medium heat. Cook patties over medium-low heat about 10 minutes or until browned on both sides.

4 Meanwhile, for sauce, combine yogurt, cucumber, mint, dill weed, black pepper, salt and hot pepper sauce, if desired, in small bowl. Serve burgers with sauce on rolls, if desired.

NUTRIENTS PER SERVING:

Calories: 124, **Total Fat:** 2g, **Saturated Fat:** 1g, **Cholesterol:** 54mg, **Sodium:** 166mg, **Carbohydrates:** 21g, **Dietary Fiber:** 1g, **Protein:** 9g
Dietary Exchange: ½ Bread/Starch, ½ Meat, 2½ Vegetable

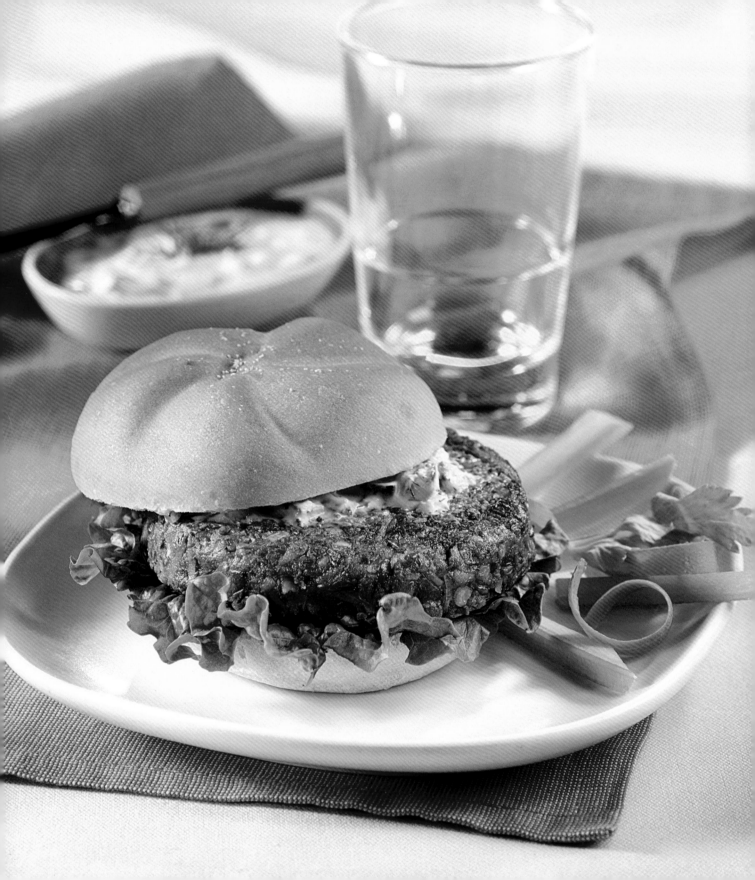

GRILLED SALMON SALAD WITH ORANGE-BASIL VINAIGRETTE

MAKES 2 SERVINGS

¼ cup frozen orange juice concentrate, thawed

1 tablespoon plus 1½ teaspoons white wine vinegar or cider vinegar

1 tablespoon chopped fresh basil *or* 1 teaspoon dried basil

1½ teaspoons olive oil

1 salmon fillet (about 8 ounces)

4 cups torn mixed greens

¾ cup sliced strawberries

10 to 12 thin cucumber slices, cut into halves

⅛ teaspoon black pepper

1. Whisk orange juice concentrate, vinegar, basil and oil in small bowl until well blended. Remove 2 tablespoons orange juice mixture; reserve remaining mixture to use as salad dressing.

2. Prepare grill for direct cooking. Spray grid with nonstick cooking spray. Grill salmon, skin side down, over medium coals 5 minutes. Turn and grill 5 minutes or until fish flakes with fork, brushing frequently with 2 tablespoons juice concentrate mixture. Cool slightly.

3. Toss together greens, strawberries and cucumber in large bowl. Place on 2 serving plates.

4. Remove skin from salmon. Break salmon into chunks; arrange on greens mixture. Drizzle with reserved orange juice mixture; sprinkle with pepper.

NUTRIENTS PER SERVING:

Calories: 283, **Total Fat:** 11g, **Saturated Fat:** 2g, **Cholesterol:** 60mg, **Sodium:** 70mg, **Carbohydrates:** 23g, **Dietary Fiber:** 3g, **Protein:** 24g
Dietary Exchange: 3 Meat, 1½ Fruit, ½ Fat

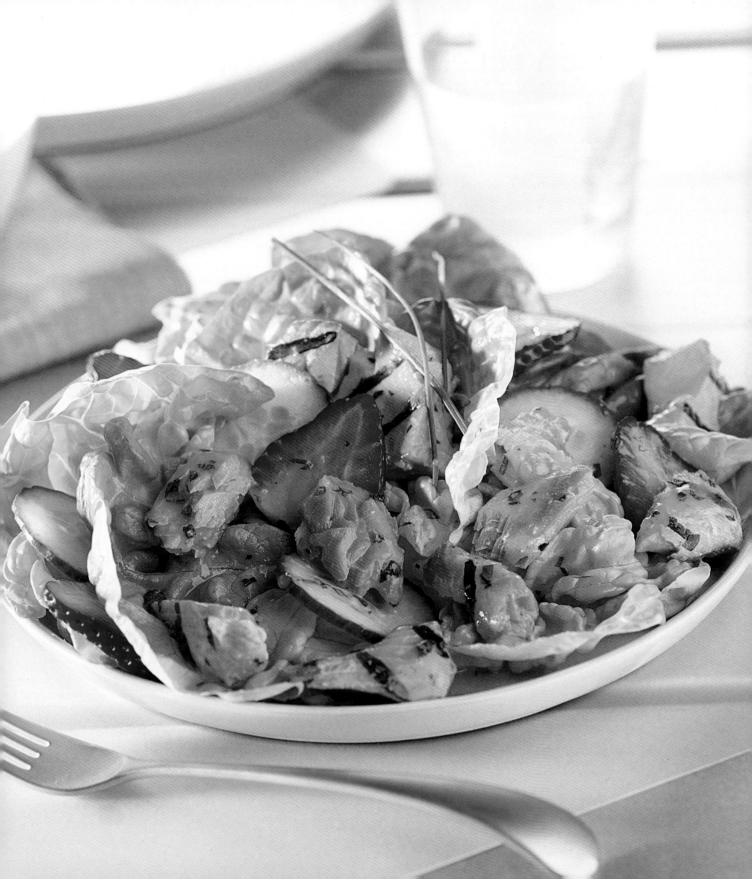

QUINOA BURRITO BOWLS

MAKES 4 SERVINGS

- 1 cup uncooked quinoa
- 2 cups water
- 2 tablespoons fresh lime juice, divided
- ¼ cup light sour cream
- 2 teaspoons vegetable oil
- 1 small onion, diced
- 1 red bell pepper, diced
- 1 clove garlic, minced
- ½ cup canned black beans, rinsed and drained
- ½ cup thawed frozen corn
- Shredded lettuce
- Lime wedges (optional)

1. Place quinoa in fine-mesh strainer; rinse well under cold running water. Bring 2 cups water to a boil in small saucepan; stir in quinoa. Reduce heat to low; cover and simmer 10 to 15 minutes or until quinoa is tender and water is absorbed. Stir in 1 tablespoon lime juice. Cover and keep warm. Combine sour cream and remaining 1 tablespoon lime juice in small bowl; set aside.

2. Meanwhile, heat oil in large skillet over medium heat. Add onion and bell pepper; cook and stir 5 minutes or until softened. Add garlic; cook 1 minute. Add black beans and corn; cook 3 to 5 minutes or until heated through.

3. Divide quinoa among 4 serving bowls; top with black bean mixture, lettuce and sour cream mixture. Garnish with lime wedges.

NUTRIENTS PER SERVING:

Calories: 258, **Total Fat:** 7g, **Saturated Fat:** 1g, **Cholesterol:** 4mg, **Sodium:** 136mg, **Carbohydrates:** 42g, **Dietary Fiber:** 6g, **Protein:** 9g
Dietary Exchange: 3 Bread/Starch, 1 Fat

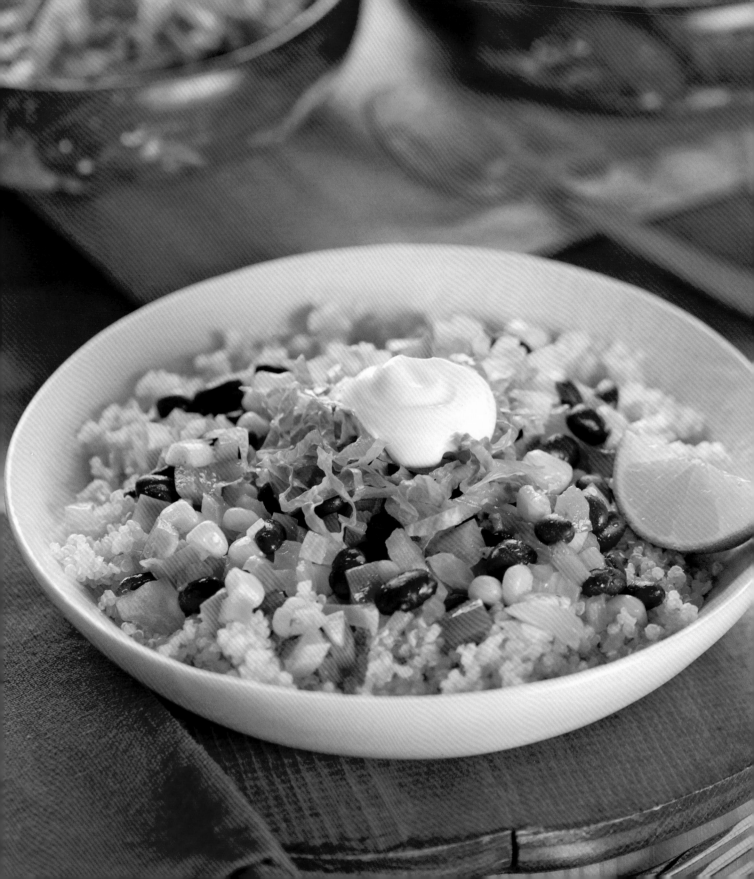

CHICKEN AND APPLE SPRING GREENS WITH POPPY SEEDS

MAKES 4 SERVINGS

---

1 package (5 ounces) spring salad greens

12 ounces cooked chicken strips

1 large Golden Delicious apple, thinly sliced

⅓ cup thinly sliced red onion

1 ounce crumbled goat cheese (optional)

¼ cup cider vinegar

2 tablespoons sugar substitute

2 tablespoons canola oil

½ teaspoon poppy seeds

¼ teaspoon salt

⅛ teaspoon red pepper flakes

---

1 Arrange equal amounts greens, chicken, apple and onion on 4 plates. Sprinkle with cheese, if desired.

2 Combine vinegar, sugar substitute, oil, poppy seeds, salt and red pepper flakes in small jar with tight-fitting lid; shake well. Drizzle dressing over salads.

NUTRIENTS PER SERVING:

Calories: 220, **Total Fat:** 9g, **Saturated Fat:** 1.5g, **Cholesterol:** 45mg, **Sodium:** 250mg, **Carbohydrates:** 10g, **Dietary Fiber:** 1g, **Protein:** 26g
Dietary Exchange: 3 Meat, 1 Vegetable, 1 Fruit, 2 Fat

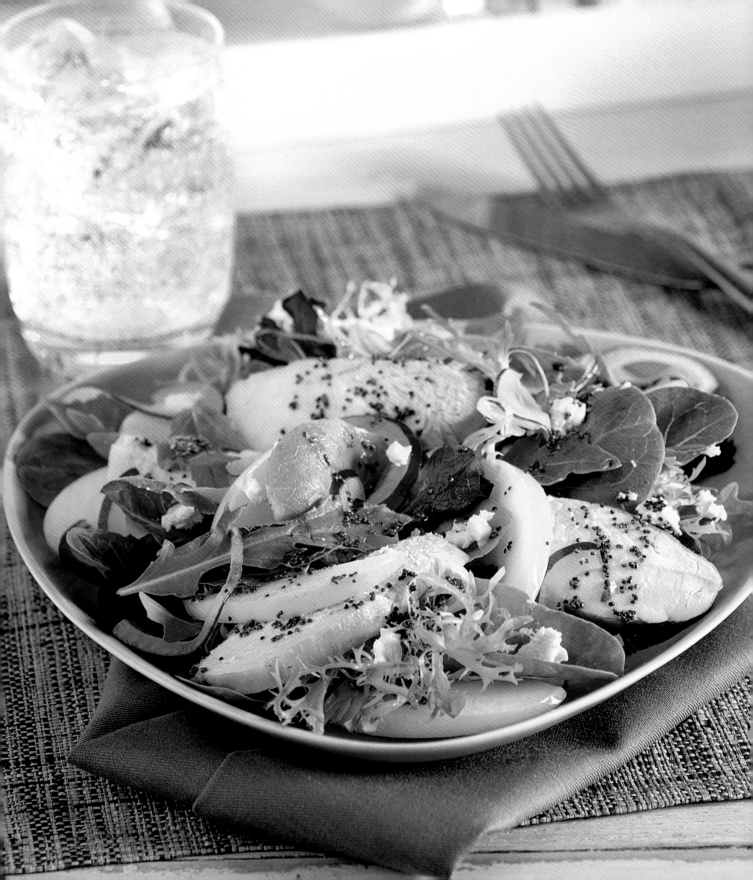

TURKEY & VEGGIE ROLL-UPS

MAKES 2 SERVINGS

---

2 tablespoons hummus, any flavor

1 (8-inch) whole wheat tortilla

¼ cup sliced baby spinach

2 slices oven-roasted turkey breast (about 1 ounce)

¼ cup thinly sliced English cucumber

1 slice (1 ounce) reduced-fat Swiss cheese

¼ cup thinly sliced carrot

Spread hummus on tortilla to within 1 inch of edge. Layer with spinach, turkey, cucumber, cheese and carrot. Roll up tortilla and filling; cut into 4 pieces.

NUTRIENTS PER SERVING:

Calories: 140, **Total Fat:** 4g, **Saturated Fat:** 1g, **Cholesterol:** 16mg, **Sodium:** 292mg, **Carbohydrates:** 14g, **Dietary Fiber:** 2g, **Protein:** 11g
Dietary Exchange: 1 Bread/Starch, 1 Meat

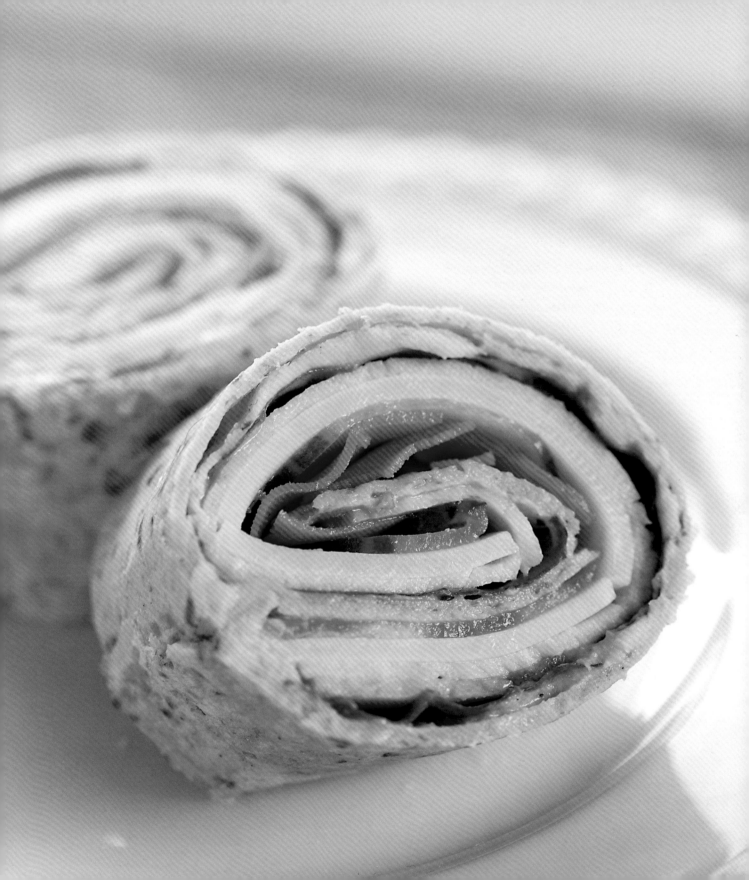

CRAB SPINACH SALAD WITH TARRAGON DRESSING

MAKES 4 SERVINGS

12 ounces coarsely flaked cooked crabmeat *or* 2 packages (6 ounces each) frozen crabmeat, thawed and drained

1 cup chopped tomatoes

1 cup sliced cucumber

⅓ cup sliced red onion

¼ cup fat-free salad dressing or mayonnaise

¼ cup reduced-fat sour cream

¼ cup chopped fresh parsley

2 tablespoons fat-free (skim) milk

2 teaspoons chopped fresh tarragon *or* ½ teaspoon dried tarragon leaves

1 clove garlic, minced

¼ teaspoon hot pepper sauce

8 cups fresh spinach

1 Combine crabmeat, tomatoes, cucumber and onion in medium bowl. Combine salad dressing, sour cream, parsley, milk, tarragon, garlic and hot pepper sauce in small bowl.

2 Line 4 salad plates with spinach. Place crabmeat mixture on spinach; drizzle with dressing.

NUTRIENTS PER SERVING:

Calories: 170, **Total Fat:** 4g, **Saturated Fat:** 1g, **Cholesterol:** 91mg, **Sodium:** 481mg, **Carbohydrates:** 14g, **Dietary Fiber:** 4g, **Protein:** 22g
Dietary Exchange: 2½ Meat, 2 Vegetable

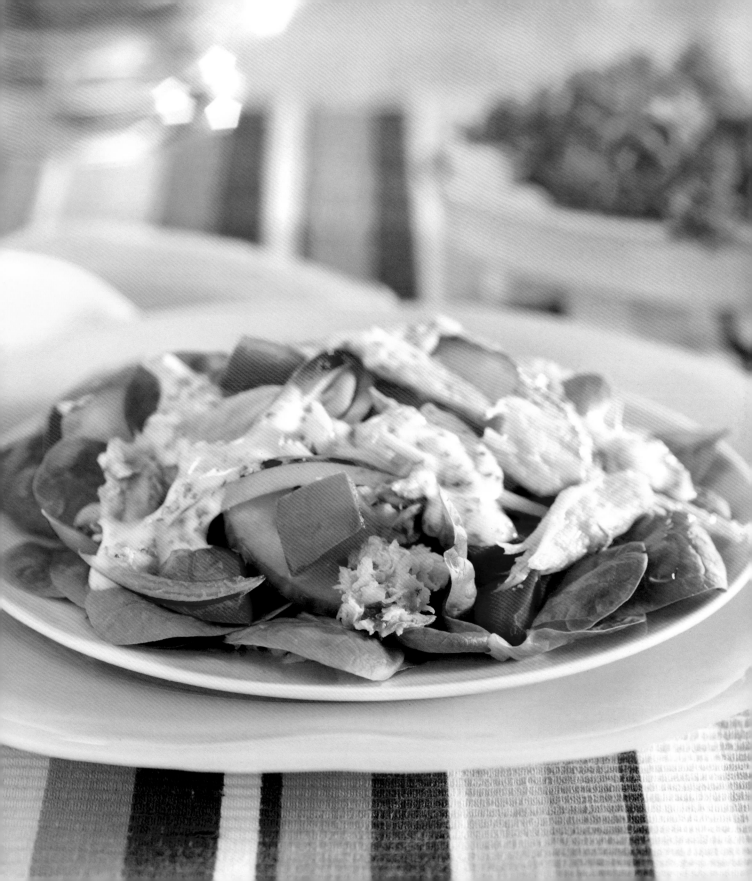

ORZO SPINACH PIE

MAKES 4 SERVINGS

⅔ **cup uncooked orzo**

1 **cup fat-free (skim) milk**

3 **egg whites**

¼ **teaspoon salt (optional)**

⅛ **teaspoon ground nutmeg**

⅛ **teaspoon black pepper**

1 **package (10 ounces) frozen chopped spinach, thawed and pressed dry**

4 **tablespoons grated Parmesan cheese, divided**

¾ **cup fresh whole wheat bread crumbs***

1 **tablespoon unsalted butter, melted**

*To make fresh bread crumbs, tear 1½ slices bread into pieces; process in food processor until coarse crumbs form.

1 Preheat oven to 375°F. Spray 9-inch pie plate with nonstick cooking spray.

2 Cook orzo according to package directions, omitting any salt. Drain.

3 Whisk milk, egg whites, salt, if desired, nutmeg and pepper in large bowl until well blended. Stir in spinach and 2 tablespoons Parmesan cheese. Add orzo; gently mix. Spoon evenly into prepared pie plate.

4 Combine bread crumbs and remaining 2 tablespoons Parmesan cheese in small bowl. Stir in butter. Sprinkle evenly over spinach mixture.

5 Bake 20 minutes or until topping is golden brown and center is set. Let stand 5 minutes before serving.

NUTRIENTS PER SERVING:

Calories: 292, **Total Fat:** 6g, **Saturated Fat:** 3g, **Cholesterol:** 13mg, **Sodium:** 399mg, **Carbohydrates:** 42g, **Dietary Fiber:** 3g, **Protein:** 15g
Dietary Exchange: 1 Bread/Starch, 1 Meat, 2 Vegetable, 1 Fat

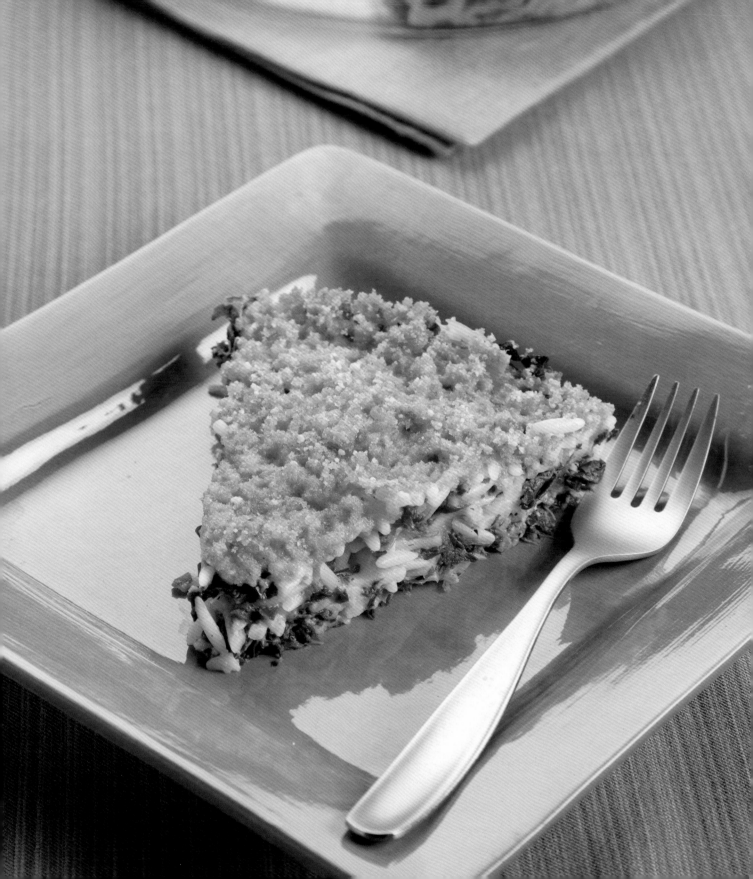

TACO SALAD

MAKES 6 SERVINGS

---

3 ounces uncooked radiatore pasta, cooked

½ cup frozen corn, thawed

½ cup chopped seeded tomato

1 can (about 4 ounces) diced mild green chiles, drained

¼ cup chopped onion

2 tablespoons sliced black olives

2 tablespoons chopped fresh cilantro

½ cup mild or medium chunky salsa

½ teaspoon chili powder

Combine pasta, corn, tomato, chiles, onion, olives and cilantro in large bowl. Combine salsa and chili powder in small bowl until well blended. Pour over pasta mixture; toss to coat. Cover; refrigerate 2 hours.

NUTRIENTS PER SERVING:

Calories: 84, **Total Fat:** 2g, **Saturated Fat:** 1g, **Cholesterol:** 1mg, **Sodium:** 471mg, **Carbohydrates:** 16g, **Dietary Fiber:** 2g, **Protein:** 3g
Dietary Exchange: 1 Bread/Starch

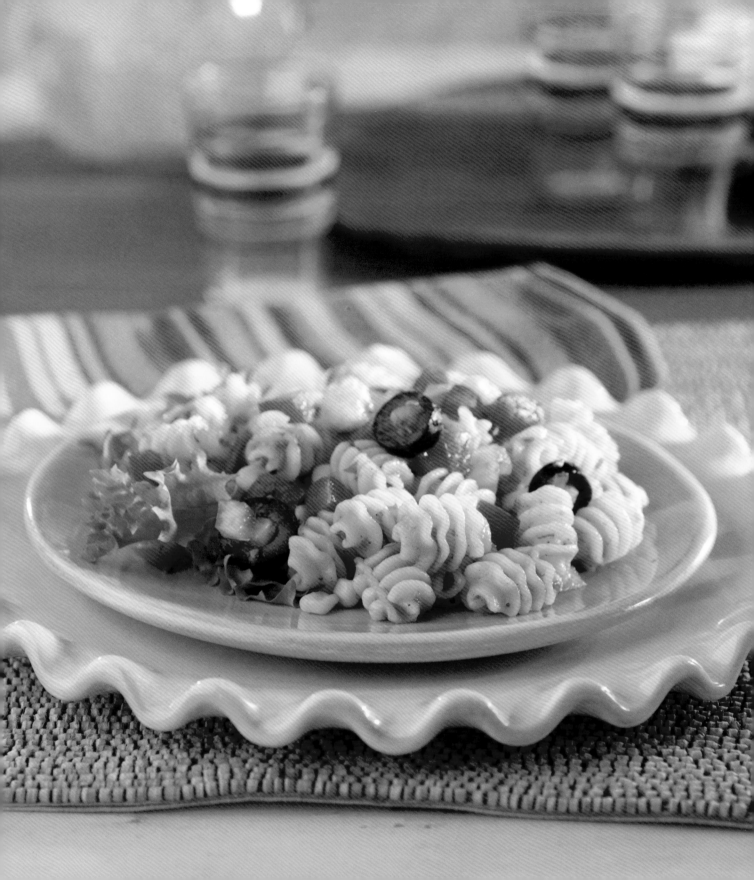

MUSHROOM TOFU BURGERS

MAKES 6 SERVINGS

7 ounces extra firm tofu

3 teaspoons olive oil, divided

1 package (8 ounces) cremini mushrooms, coarsely chopped

½ medium onion, coarsely chopped

1 clove garlic, minced

1 cup old-fashioned oats

⅓ cup finely chopped walnuts

1 egg

½ teaspoon salt

½ teaspoon onion powder

¼ teaspoon dried thyme

6 light multi-grain English muffins, split and toasted

Lettuce, tomato and red onion slices (optional)

1 Crumble tofu; spread on small baking sheet or freezer-safe plate. Freeze 1 hour or until firm.

2 Heat 1 teaspoon oil in large nonstick skillet over medium heat. Add mushrooms, onion and garlic; cook and stir 10 minutes or until mushrooms are tender and any water from mushrooms has evaporated. Remove from heat; cool slightly.

3 Combine mushroom mixture, tofu, oats, walnuts, egg, salt, onion powder and thyme in food processor or blender; process until combined. (Some tofu pieces may remain). Shape mixture into 6 (⅓-cup) patties.

4 Heat 1 teaspoon oil in same skillet over medium-low heat. Working in batches, cook patties 5 minutes per side. Repeat with remaining oil and patties. Serve on English muffins with lettuce, tomato and red onion, if desired.

NUTRIENTS PER SERVING:

Calories: 254, **Total Fat:** 10g, **Saturated Fat:** 1g, **Cholesterol:** 31mg, **Sodium:** 469mg, **Carbohydrates:** 37g, **Dietary Fiber:** 9g, **Protein:** 13g
Dietary Exchange: 2½ Bread/Starch, 1 Meat, 1 Fat

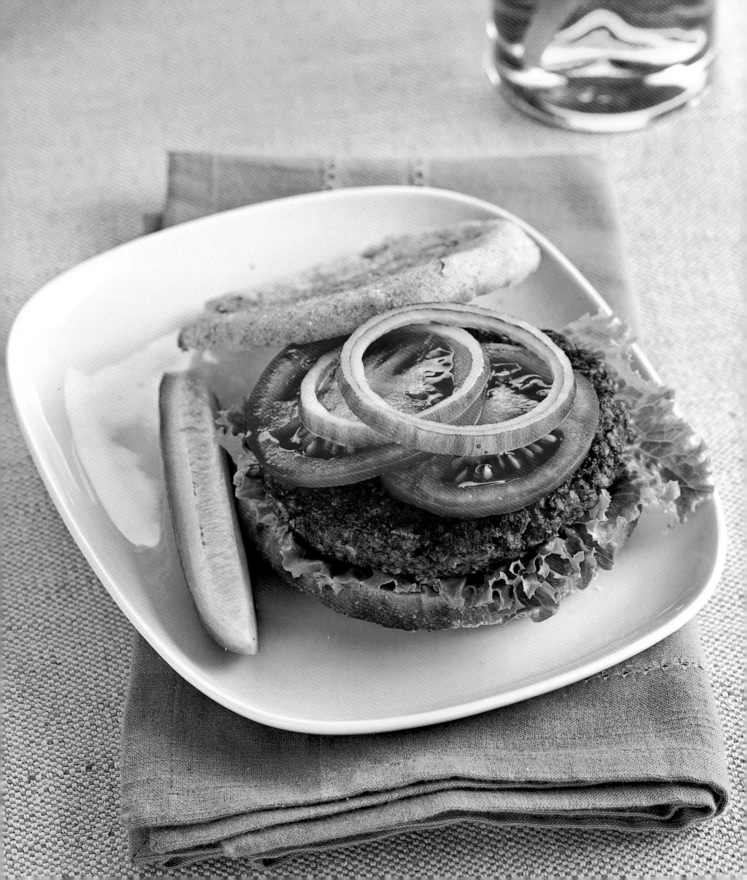

CHICKEN AND SPINACH SALAD

MAKES 4 SERVINGS

¾ pound chicken tenders

4 cups shredded stemmed spinach

2 cups washed and torn romaine lettuce

1 large grapefruit, peeled and sectioned

8 thin slices red onion, separated into rings

2 tablespoons crumbled blue cheese

½ cup frozen citrus blend concentrate, thawed

¼ cup prepared fat-free Italian salad dressing

1 Cut chicken into 2×½-inch strips. Spray large nonstick skillet with nonstick cooking spray; heat over medium heat. Add chicken; cook and stir 5 minutes or until no longer pink in center. Remove from skillet.

2 Divide spinach, lettuce, grapefruit, onion, cheese and chicken among 4 salad plates. Combine citrus blend concentrate and Italian dressing in small bowl; drizzle over salads.

NUTRIENTS PER SERVING:

Calories: 218, **Total Fat:** 4g, **Saturated Fat:** 1g, **Cholesterol:** 55mg, **Sodium:** 361mg, **Carbohydrates:** 23g, **Dietary Fiber:** 3g, **Protein:** 23g
Dietary Exchange: 2½ Meat, 2 Vegetable, 1 Fruit

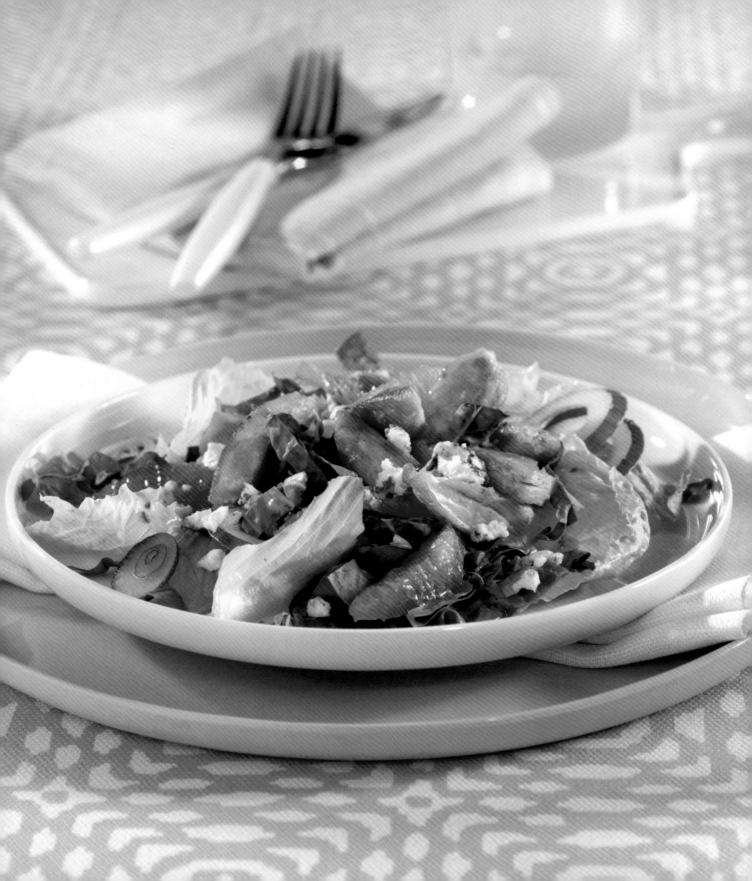

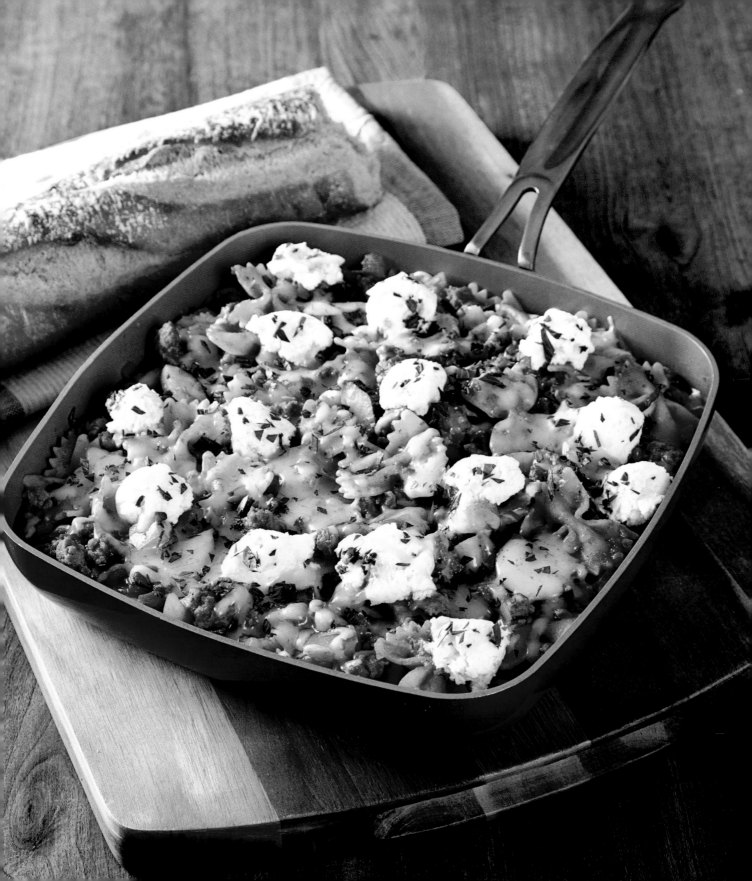

Mainstay Dinners

SKILLET LASAGNA WITH VEGETABLES

MAKES 6 SERVINGS

½ pound hot Italian turkey sausage, casings removed

½ pound 93% lean ground turkey

2 stalks celery, sliced

⅓ cup chopped onion

2 cups marinara sauce

1⅓ cups water

4 ounces uncooked bowtie (farfalle) pasta

1 medium zucchini, halved lengthwise, then cut crosswise into ½-inch slices (2 cups)

¾ cup chopped green or yellow bell pepper

½ cup (2 ounces) shredded part-skim mozzarella cheese

½ cup reduced-fat ricotta cheese

2 tablespoons finely grated Parmesan cheese

1 Heat large skillet over medium-high heat. Add sausage, ground turkey, celery and onion; cook and stir 6 to 8 minutes or until turkey is no longer pink. Stir in marinara sauce and water; bring to a boil. Stir in pasta. Reduce heat to medium-low; cover and simmer 12 minutes.

2 Stir in zucchini and bell pepper; cover and simmer 2 minutes. Uncover and simmer 4 to 6 minutes or until vegetables are crisp-tender.

3 Sprinkle with mozzarella. Combine ricotta and Parmesan cheese in small bowl; stir to blend. Drop by rounded teaspoonfuls on top of mixture in skillet. Remove from heat; cover and let stand 10 minutes.

NUTRIENTS PER SERVING:

Calories: 300, **Total Fat:** 11g, **Saturated Fat:** 2.5g, **Cholesterol:** 45mg, **Sodium:** 750mg, **Carbohydrates:** 24g, **Dietary Fiber:** 3g, **Protein:** 25g
Dietary Exchange: 1 Bread/Starch, 2½ Meat, ½ Fat

PORK AND PLUM KABOBS

MAKES 4 SERVINGS

¾ pound boneless pork loin chops (1 inch thick), trimmed and cut into 1-inch pieces

1½ teaspoons ground cumin

½ teaspoon ground cinnamon

¼ teaspoon salt

¼ teaspoon garlic powder

¼ teaspoon ground red pepper

¼ cup sliced green onions

¼ cup raspberry fruit spread

1 tablespoon orange juice

3 plums or nectarines, pitted and cut into wedges

1 Place pork in large resealable food storage bag. Combine cumin, cinnamon, salt, garlic powder and ground red pepper in small bowl; pour over pork. Seal bag; shake to coat meat with spices.

2 Combine green onions, fruit spread and orange juice in small bowl; set aside.

3 Prepare grill for direct cooking. Alternately thread pork and plum wedges onto 8 skewers.* Grill kabobs over medium heat 12 to 14 minutes or until meat is cooked through, turning once. Brush frequently with raspberry mixture during last 5 minutes of grilling.

*If using wooden skewers, soak in cool water 20 to 30 minutes to prevent burning.

SERVING SUGGESTION: A crisp, cool salad makes a great accompaniment to these sweet grilled kabobs.

NUTRIENTS PER SERVING:

Calories: 191, **Total Fat:** 5g, **Saturated Fat:** 2g, **Cholesterol:** 53mg, **Sodium:** 183mg, **Carbohydrates:** 17g, **Dietary Fiber:** 1g, **Protein:** 19g
Dietary Exchange: 3 Meat, 1 Fruit

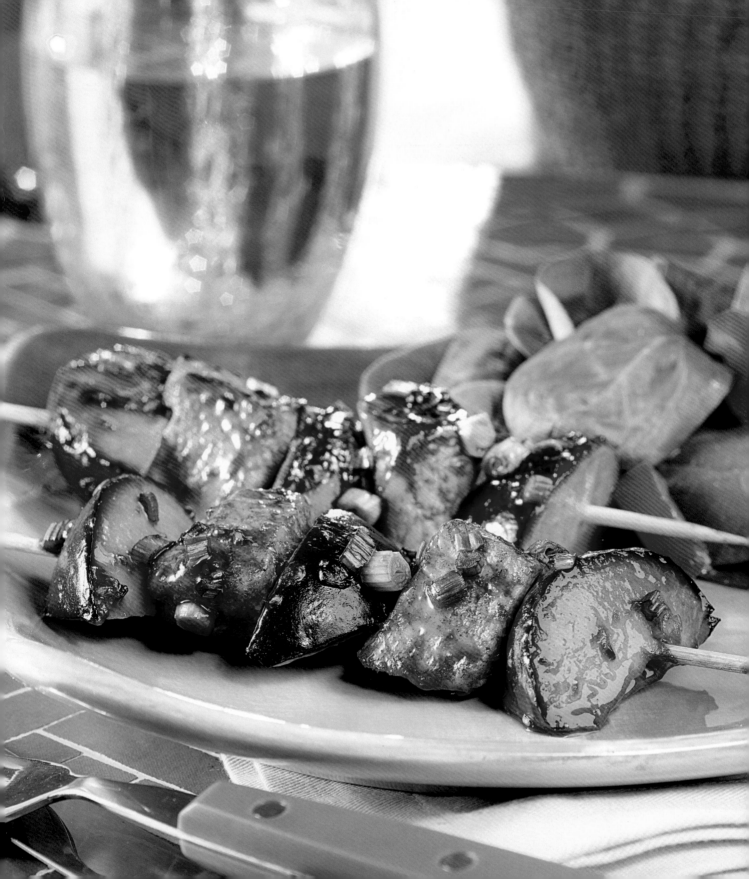

CHICKEN PICCATA

MAKES 4 SERVINGS

3 tablespoons all-purpose flour

½ teaspoon salt

¼ teaspoon black pepper

4 boneless skinless chicken breasts
(4 ounces each)

2 teaspoons olive oil

1 teaspoon butter

2 cloves garlic, minced

¾ cup fat-free reduced-sodium
chicken broth

1 tablespoon fresh lemon juice

2 tablespoons chopped fresh Italian
parsley

1 tablespoon capers, drained

1 Combine flour, salt and pepper in shallow dish. Reserve 1 tablespoon flour
mixture for sauce.

2 Pound chicken to ½-inch thickness between sheets of waxed paper with flat side
of meat mallet or rolling pin. Coat chicken with remaining flour mixture, shaking
off excess.

3 Heat oil and butter in large nonstick skillet over medium heat. Add chicken; cook
4 to 5 minutes per side or until no longer pink in center. Transfer to serving platter;
cover loosely with foil.

4 Add garlic to skillet; cook and stir 1 minute. Add reserved flour mixture; cook and
stir 1 minute. Add broth and lemon juice; cook 2 minutes or until sauce thickens,
stirring frequently. Stir in parsley and capers; spoon sauce over chicken.

NUTRIENTS PER SERVING:

Calories: 194, **Total Fat:** 6g, **Saturated Fat:** 2g, **Cholesterol:** 71mg, **Sodium:** 473mg,
Carbohydrates: 5g, **Dietary Fiber:** 1g, **Protein:** 27g
Dietary Exchange: ½ Bread/Starch, 3 Meat

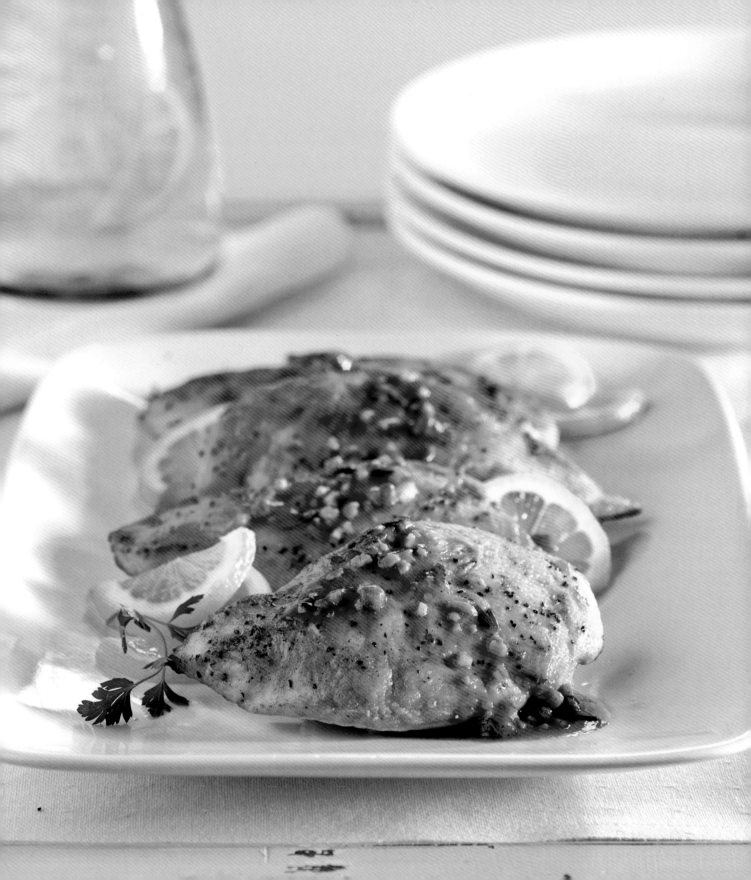

ZESTY SKILLET PORK CHOPS

MAKES 4 SERVINGS

1 teaspoon chili powder

½ teaspoon salt, divided

4 lean boneless pork chops (about 1¼ pounds), well trimmed

2 cups diced tomatoes

1 cup chopped green, red or yellow bell pepper

¾ cup thinly sliced celery

½ cup chopped onion

1 teaspoon dried thyme

1 tablespoon hot pepper sauce

2 tablespoons finely chopped fresh parsley

1 Rub chili powder and ¼ teaspoon salt evenly over one side of pork chops.

2 Combine tomatoes, bell peppers, celery, onion, thyme and hot pepper sauce in medium bowl; mix well.

3 Lightly spray large nonstick skillet with nonstick cooking spray; heat over medium-high heat. Add pork, seasoned side down; cook 1 minute. Turn pork. Top with tomato mixture; bring to a boil. Reduce heat to low. Cover; cook 25 minutes or until pork is tender and tomato mixture has thickened.

4 Remove pork to serving plates. Bring tomato mixture to a boil over high heat; cook 2 minutes or until most liquid has evaporated. Remove from heat; stir in parsley and remaining ¼ teaspoon salt. Spoon sauce over pork.

NUTRIENTS PER SERVING:

Calories: 172, **Total Fat:** 7g, **Saturated Fat:** 2g, **Cholesterol:** 49mg, **Sodium:** 387mg, **Carbohydrates:** 9g, **Dietary Fiber:** 3g, **Protein:** 20g
Dietary Exchange: 2 Meat, 2 Vegetable

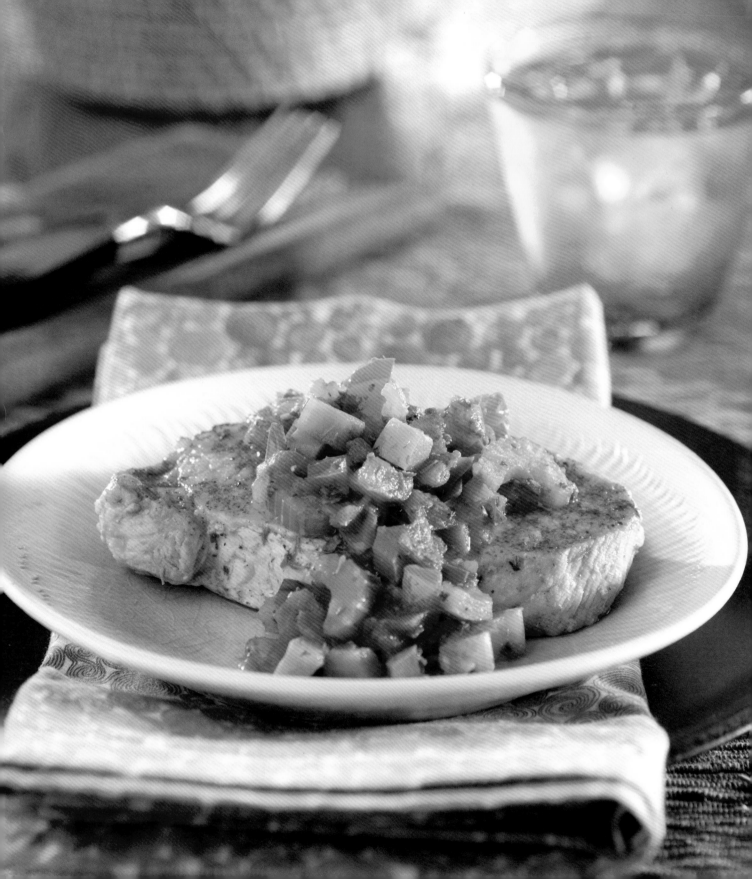

SCALLOP AND ARTICHOKE HEART CASSEROLE

MAKES 4 SERVINGS

1 package (9 ounces) frozen artichoke hearts, cooked and drained

1 pound scallops

1 teaspoon canola or vegetable oil

¼ cup chopped red bell pepper

¼ cup sliced green onions

¼ cup all-purpose flour

2 cups low-fat (1%) milk

1 teaspoon dried tarragon

¼ teaspoon salt

¼ teaspoon white pepper

1 tablespoon chopped fresh parsley

Pinch paprika

1 Preheat oven to 350°F.

2 Cut large artichoke hearts lengthwise into halves; arrange in even layer in 8-inch square baking dish.

3 Rinse scallops; pat dry with paper towel. If scallops are large, cut into halves. Arrange scallops evenly over artichokes.

4 Heat oil in medium saucepan over medium-low heat. Add bell pepper and green onions; cook and stir 5 minutes or until tender. Stir in flour. Gradually stir in milk until smooth. Add tarragon, salt and white pepper; cook and stir over medium heat 10 minutes or until sauce boils and thickens. Pour sauce over scallops.

5 Bake, uncovered, 25 minutes or until casserole is bubbly and scallops are opaque. Sprinkle with parsley and paprika before serving.

TIP: White pepper is a mild version of the common black pepper. They both originate from the same berries, which are called peppercorns. White pepper helps to maintain consistent color in light foods.

NUTRIENTS PER SERVING:

Calories: 227, **Total Fat:** 4g, **Saturated Fat:** 1g, **Cholesterol:** 43mg, **Sodium:** 438mg, **Carbohydrates:** 23g, **Dietary Fiber:** 4g, **Protein:** 26g
Dietary Exchange: 2½ Meat, 2 Vegetable, ½ Milk

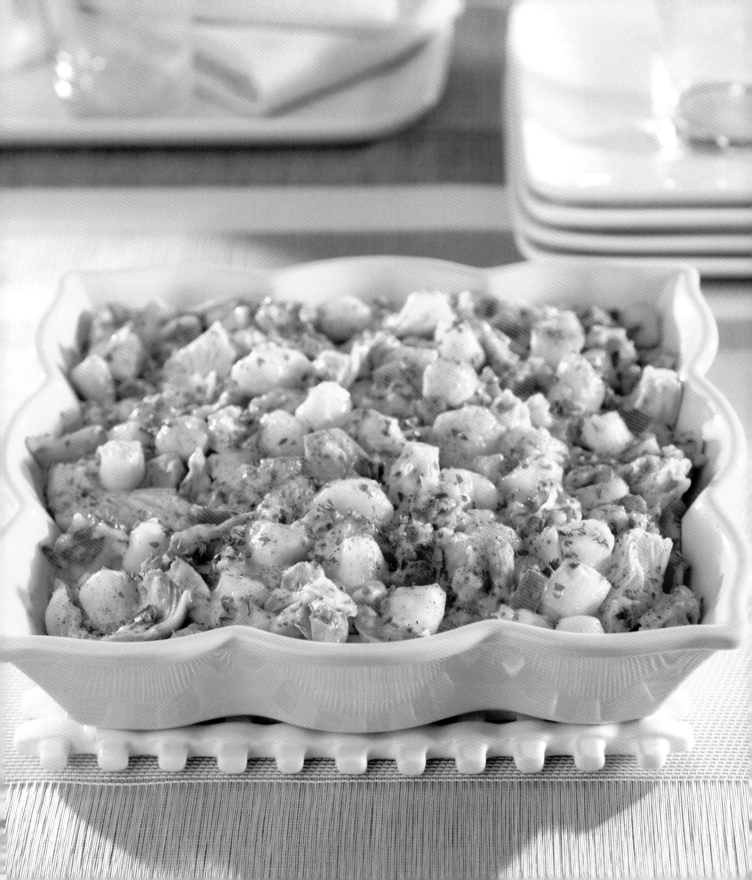

EASY MOO SHU PORK

MAKES 2 SERVINGS

---

7 ounces pork tenderloin, sliced

4 green onions, cut into ½-inch pieces

1½ cups packaged coleslaw mix

2 tablespoons hoisin sauce or Asian plum sauce

4 (8-inch) fat-free flour tortillas, warmed

---

1 Spray large nonstick skillet with nonstick cooking spray; heat over medium-high heat. Add pork and green onions; stir-fry 2 to 3 minutes or until pork is barely pink in center. Stir in coleslaw mix and hoisin sauce.

2 Spoon pork mixture onto tortillas. Roll up tortillas, folding in sides to enclose filling.

NOTE: To warm tortillas, stack and wrap loosely in plastic wrap. Microwave on HIGH 15 to 20 seconds or until warm and pliable.

NUTRIENTS PER SERVING:

Calories: 293, **Total Fat:** 4g, **Saturated Fat:** 1g, **Cholesterol:** 58mg, **Sodium:** 672mg, **Carbohydrates:** 37g, **Dietary Fiber:** 14g, **Protein:** 26g
Dietary Exchange: 2 Bread/Starch, 2 Meat, 1 Vegetable

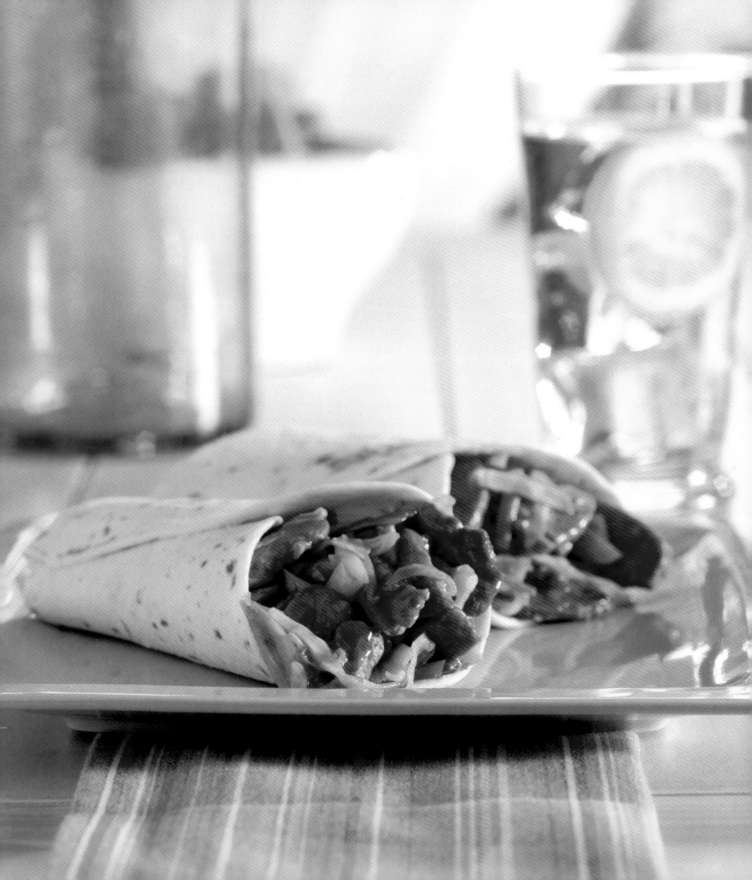

SOUTHWEST ROASTED SALMON & CORN

MAKES 2 SERVINGS

---

2 medium ears fresh corn, unhusked

1 salmon fillet (6 ounces), cut in half

1 tablespoon plus 1 teaspoon lime juice, divided

1 clove garlic, minced

½ teaspoon chili powder

¼ teaspoon ground cumin

¼ teaspoon dried oregano

⅛ teaspoon salt, divided

⅛ teaspoon black pepper

2 teaspoons margarine or butter, melted

2 teaspoons minced fresh cilantro

---

1 Pull back husks from each ear of corn, leaving attached. Discard silk. Bring husks back up over each ear. Soak corn in cold water 20 minutes.

2 Preheat oven to 400°F. Spray shallow 1-quart baking dish with nonstick cooking spray. Place salmon, skin side down, in prepared dish. Pour 1 tablespoon lime juice over fish. Marinate at room temperature 15 minutes.

3 Combine garlic, chili powder, cumin, oregano, half of salt and pepper in small bowl. Pat salmon lightly with paper towel; rub garlic mixture over salmon.

4 Remove corn from water. Place corn directly on oven rack. Roast 10 minutes; turn. Place salmon in baking dish next to corn. Roast 15 minutes or until salmon is opaque and flakes when tested with fork and corn is tender.

5 Combine margarine, cilantro, remaining 1 teaspoon lime juice and remaining salt in small bowl. Remove husks from corn. Brush over corn. Serve corn with salmon.

TIP: Corn can also be cooked in boiling water. Omit steps 1 and 4. Husk the corn and place in a large pot of boiling water. Cover; remove from heat and let stand for 10 minutes. Drain and brush with cilantro mixture as directed.

NUTRIENTS PER SERVING:

Calories: 186, **Total Fat:** 6g, **Saturated Fat:** 1g, **Cholesterol:** 43mg, **Sodium:** 243mg, **Carbohydrates:** 16g, **Dietary Fiber:** 2g, **Protein:** 19g
Dietary Exchange: 1 Bread/Starch, 2 Meat

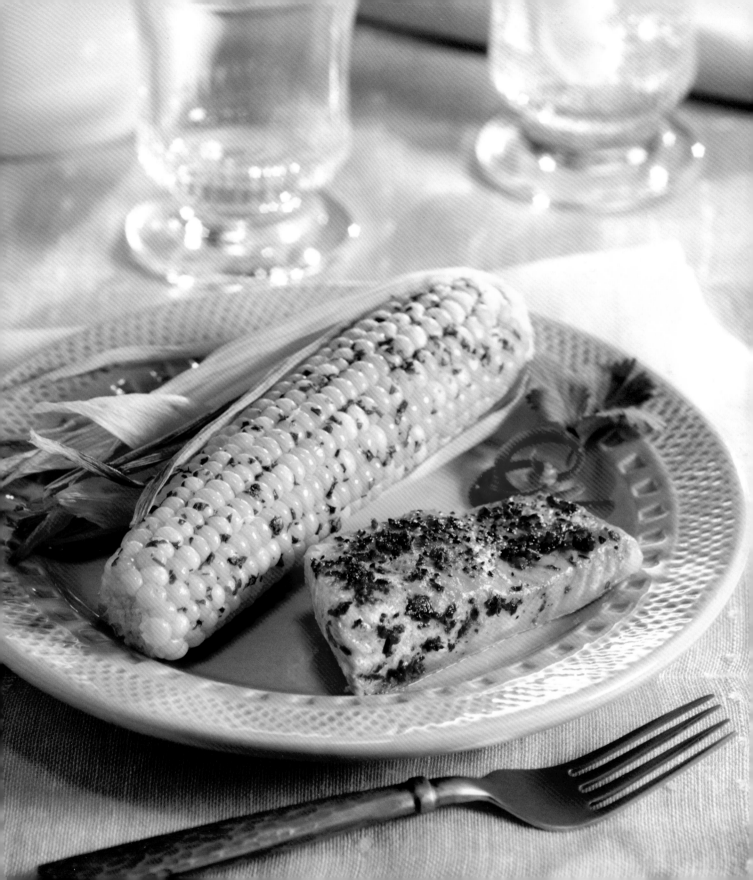

TURKEY AND VEGGIE MEATBALLS WITH FENNEL

MAKES 6 SERVINGS

- **1** pound lean ground turkey
- **½** cup finely chopped green onions
- **½** cup finely chopped green bell pepper
- **⅓** cup old-fashioned oats
- **¼** cup shredded carrot
- **¼** cup grated Parmesan cheese
- **2** egg whites

- **2** cloves garlic, minced
- **½** teaspoon Italian seasoning
- **¼** teaspoon fennel seeds
- **¼** teaspoon salt
- **⅛** teaspoon red pepper flakes (optional)
- **1** teaspoon extra virgin olive oil

1. Combine all ingredients except oil in large bowl; mix well. Shape into 36 (1-inch) balls.

2. Heat oil in large nonstick skillet over medium-high heat. Add meatballs; cook 11 minutes or until no longer pink in center, turning frequently. Use fork and spoon for easy turning. Serve immediately or cool and freeze.*

To freeze, cool completely and place in gallon-size resealable food storage bag. Release any excess air from bag and seal. Freeze bag flat for easier storage and faster thawing. This will also allow you to remove as many meatballs as needed without them sticking together. To reheat, place meatballs in a 12×8-inch microwavable dish and cook on HIGH 20 to 30 seconds or until hot.

SERVING SUGGESTION: Top with a lower-sodium meatless marinara sauce.

NUTRIENTS PER SERVING:

Calories: 159, **Total Fat:** 7g, **Saturated Fat:** 2g, **Cholesterol:** 50mg, **Sodium:** 225mg, **Carbohydrates:** 5g, **Dietary Fiber:** 1g, **Protein:** 19g
Dietary Exchange: 2 Meat, 1 Vegetable, ½ Fat

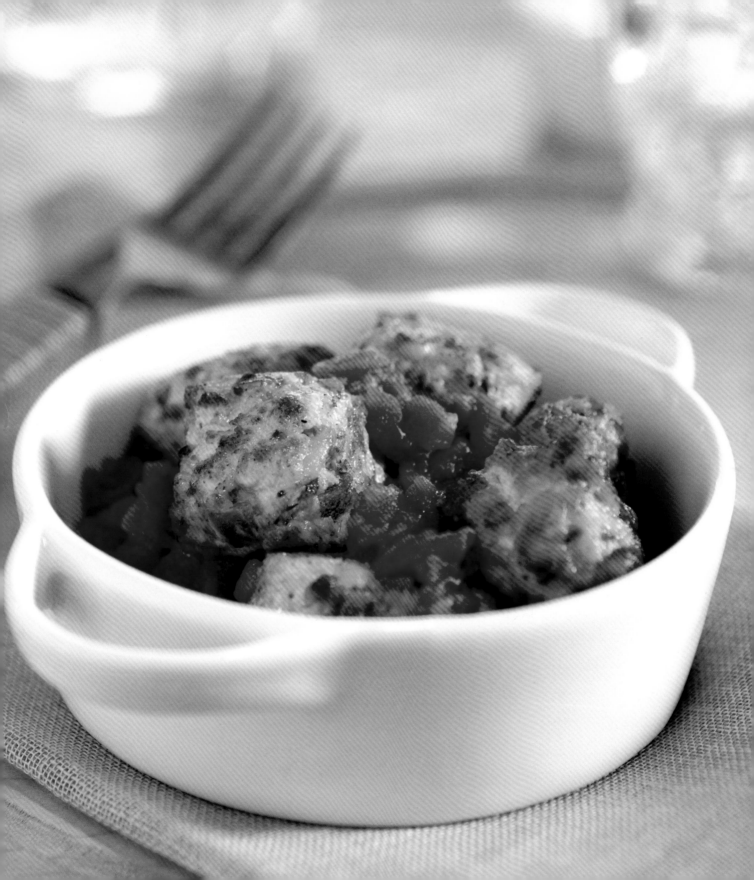

GREEK-STYLE BEEF KABOBS

MAKES 4 SERVINGS

1 pound boneless beef top sirloin steak (1 inch thick), cut into 16 pieces

¼ cup fat-free Italian salad dressing

3 tablespoons fresh lemon juice, divided

1 tablespoon dried oregano

1 tablespoon Worcestershire sauce

2 teaspoons dried basil

1 teaspoon grated lemon peel

⅛ teaspoon red pepper flakes

1 large green bell pepper, cut into 16 pieces

16 cherry tomatoes

2 teaspoons olive oil

⅛ teaspoon salt

1 Combine beef, salad dressing, 2 tablespoons lemon juice, oregano, Worcestershire sauce, basil, lemon peel and red pepper flakes in large resealable food storage bag. Seal bag; turn to coat. Marinate in refrigerator at least 8 hours or overnight, turning occasionally.

2 Preheat broiler. Remove beef from marinade; reserve marinade. Thread 4 (10-inch) skewers with beef, alternating with bell pepper and tomatoes. Spray rimmed baking sheet or broiler pan with nonstick cooking spray. Brush kabobs with marinade; place on baking sheet. Discard remaining marinade. Broil kabobs 3 minutes. Turn over; broil 2 minutes or until desired doneness is reached. Remove skewers to serving platter.

3 Add remaining 1 tablespoon lemon juice, oil and salt to pan drippings on baking sheet; stir well, scraping bottom of pan with flat spatula. Pour juices over kabobs.

NUTRIENTS PER SERVING:

Calories: 193, **Total Fat:** 8g, **Saturated Fat:** 2g, **Cholesterol:** 69mg, **Sodium:** 159mg, **Carbohydrates:** 5g, **Dietary Fiber:** 1g, **Protein:** 25g
Dietary Exchange: 3 Meat, 1 Vegetable

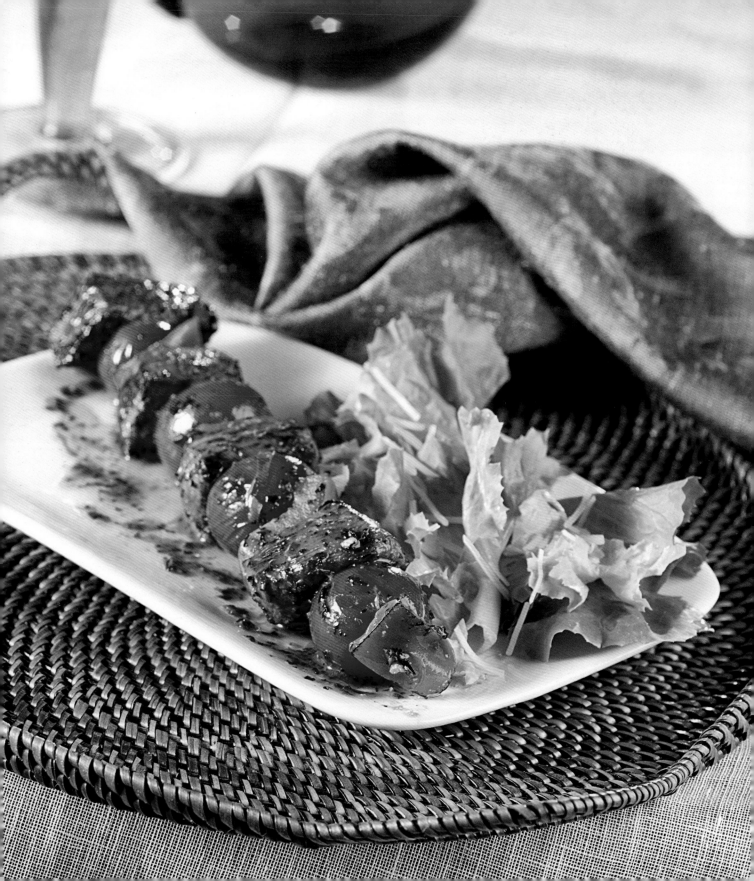

GRILLED CHICKEN, RICE & VEGGIES

MAKES 2 SERVINGS

---

2 boneless skinless chicken breasts (about 3 ounces each)

6 tablespoons reduced-fat Italian salad dressing, divided

1 cup fat-free reduced-sodium chicken broth

½ cup uncooked rice

1 cup frozen broccoli and carrot blend, thawed

---

1 Place chicken and 2 tablespoons salad dressing in large resealable food storage bag. Seal bag; turn to coat. Marinate in refrigerator 1 hour.

2 Remove chicken from marinade; discard marinade. Grill chicken over medium-hot coals 8 to 10 minutes or until chicken is no longer pink in center.

3 Meanwhile, bring broth to a boil in small saucepan; add rice. Cover; reduce heat and simmer 15 minutes, stirring in vegetables during last 5 minutes of cooking. Remove from heat and stir in remaining 4 tablespoons dressing. Serve with chicken.

NUTRIENTS PER SERVING:

Calories: 268, **Total Fat:** 7g, **Saturated Fat:** 1g, **Cholesterol:** 54mg, **Sodium:** 516mg, **Carbohydrates:** 25g, **Dietary Fiber:** 4g, **Protein:** 26g
Dietary Exchange: 1½ Bread/Starch, 2 Meat, 1 Vegetable

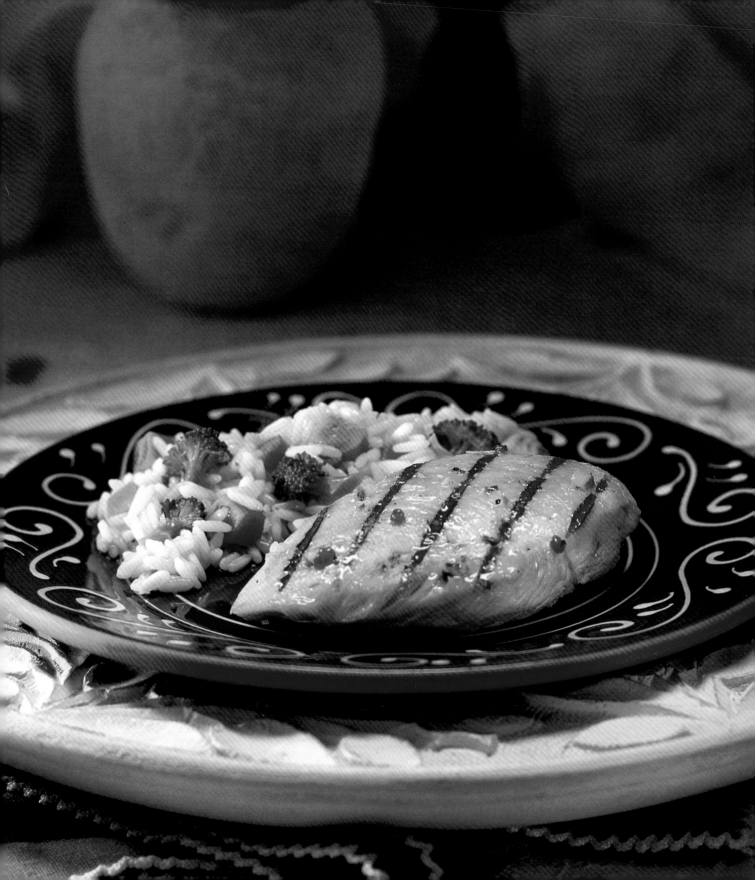

SHRIMP AND PINEAPPLE KABOBS

MAKES 4 SERVINGS

½ pound medium raw shrimp, peeled and deveined (with tails on)

½ cup pineapple juice

¼ teaspoon garlic powder

12 chunks canned pineapple

1 green bell pepper, cut into 1-inch pieces

¼ cup prepared chili sauce

1. Combine shrimp, juice and garlic powder in medium bowl; toss to coat. Marinate in refrigerator 30 minutes. Drain shrimp; discard marinade.

2. Alternately thread pineapple, bell pepper and shrimp onto 4 (10-inch) skewers. Brush with chili sauce. Grill 4 inches from heat 5 minutes or until shrimp are opaque, turning once and basting with chili sauce.

NUTRIENTS PER SERVING:

Calories: 100, **Total Fat:** 1g, **Saturated Fat:** 1g, **Cholesterol:** 87mg, **Sodium:** 302mg, **Carbohydrates:** 14g, **Dietary Fiber:** 1g, **Protein:** 10g
Dietary Exchange: 1 Meat, 1 Vegetable, 1 Fruit

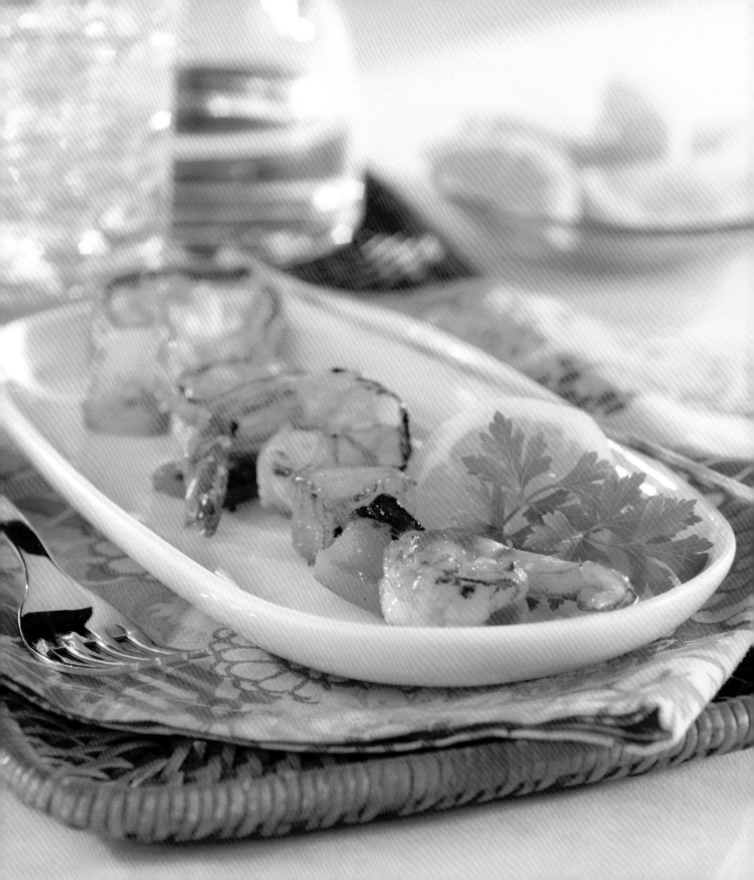

CHICKEN MIRABELLA

MAKES 4 SERVINGS

4 boneless skinless chicken breasts (about 4 ounces each)

½ cup pitted prunes

½ cup assorted pitted olives (black, green and/or a combination)

¼ cup light white grape juice or dry white wine

2 tablespoons olive oil

1 tablespoon capers

1 tablespoon red wine vinegar

1 teaspoon dried oregano

1 clove garlic, minced

½ teaspoon chopped fresh parsley, plus additional for garnish

2 teaspoons packed brown sugar

1 Preheat oven to 350°F.

2 Place chicken in 8-inch baking dish. Combine prunes, olives, grape juice, oil, capers, vinegar, oregano, garlic and ½ teaspoon parsley in medium bowl. Pour evenly over chicken. Sprinkle with brown sugar.

3 Bake 25 to 30 minutes or until chicken is no longer pink in center, basting with sauce halfway through cooking. Garnish with additional parsley.

TIP: For more intense flavor, marinate chicken at least 8 hours or overnight and sprinkle with brown sugar just before baking.

NUTRIENTS PER SERVING:

Calories: 280, **Total Fat:** 11g, **Saturated Fat:** 2g, **Cholesterol:** 72mg, **Sodium:** 291mg, **Carbohydrates:** 20g, **Dietary Fiber:** 2g, **Protein:** 25g
Dietary Exchange: 3 Meat, 1 Fruit, 1 Fat

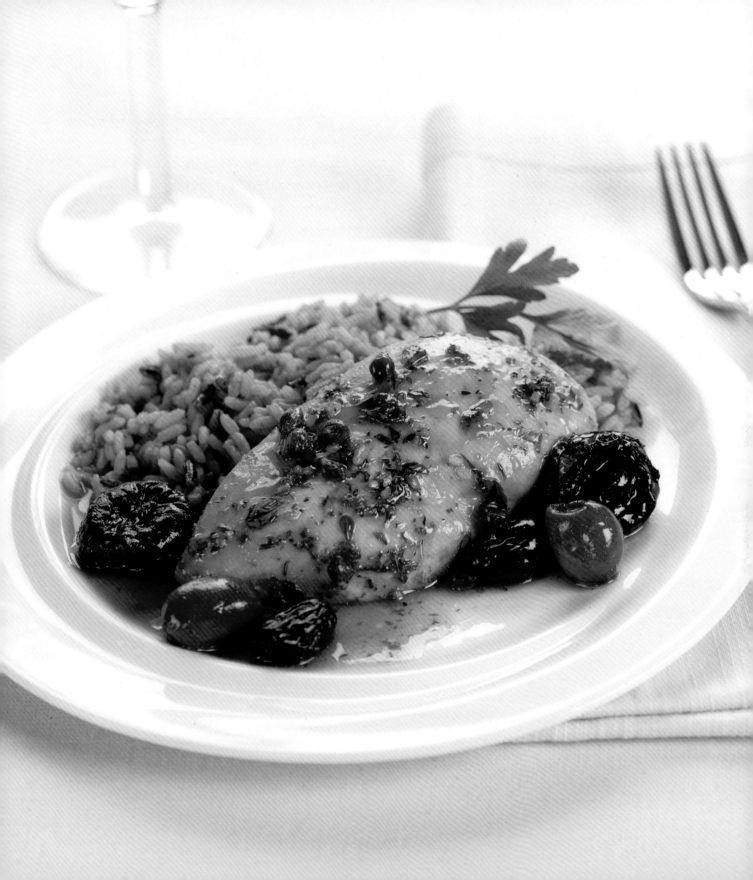

MINI MEATLOAVES

MAKES 6 SERVINGS

---

3 tablespoons ketchup

1 tablespoon balsamic vinegar

1 tablespoon olive oil

1½ cups finely chopped onion

1½ cups finely chopped mushrooms

1½ cups chopped baby spinach

1½ pounds extra lean ground sirloin

¾ cup old-fashioned oats

2 egg whites

½ teaspoon salt

½ teaspoon black pepper

---

1. Preheat oven to 375°F. Spray 6 mini (4¼×2½-inch) loaf pans with nonstick cooking spray. Whisk ketchup and vinegar in small bowl until smooth and well blended; set aside.

2. Heat oil in large skillet over medium heat. Add onion, mushrooms and spinach; cook and stir 8 minutes or until tender. Remove to large bowl. Let stand until cool enough to handle.

3. Add beef, oats, egg whites, salt and pepper to vegetables; mix well. Divide mixture evenly among prepared pans. Brush half of ketchup mixture evenly over loaves.

4. Bake 15 minutes. Brush with remaining ketchup mixture. Bake 5 minutes or until cooked through (160°F).

NUTRIENTS PER SERVING:

Calories: 270, **Total Fat:** 11g, **Saturated Fat:** 3g, **Cholesterol:** 62mg, **Sodium:** 362mg, **Carbohydrates:** 14g, **Dietary Fiber:** 2g, **Protein:** 28g
Dietary Exchange: 1 Bread/Starch, 3½ Meat

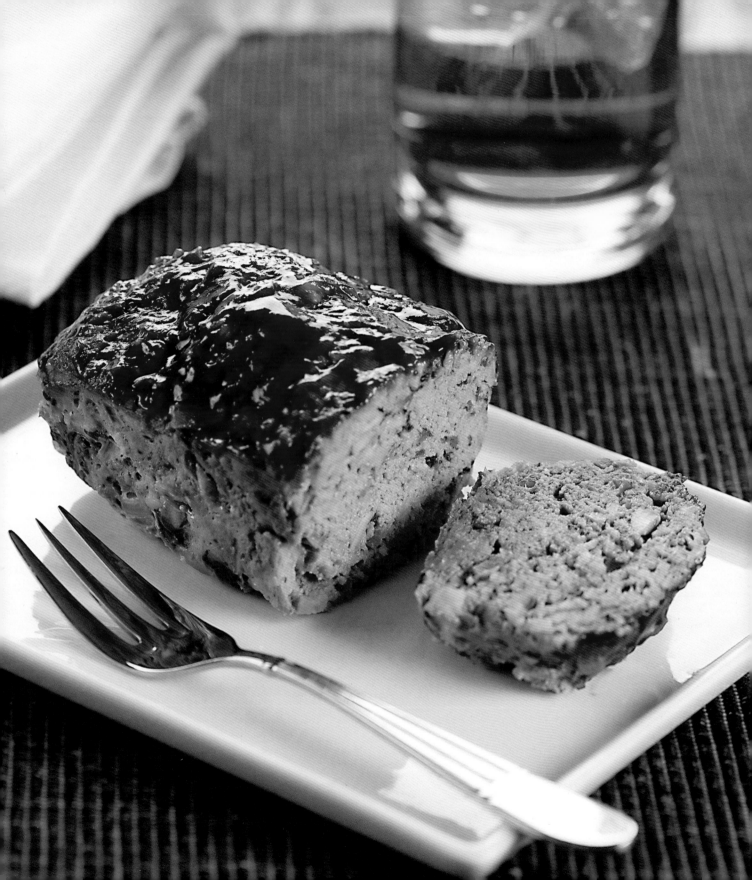

SKILLET FISH WITH LEMON TARRAGON "BUTTER"

MAKES 2 SERVINGS

2 teaspoons butter

4 teaspoons lemon juice, divided

½ teaspoon grated lemon peel

¼ teaspoon prepared mustard

¼ teaspoon dried tarragon

⅛ teaspoon salt

2 lean white fish fillets (4 ounces each),* rinsed and patted dry

¼ teaspoon paprika

Cod, orange roughy, flounder, haddock, halibut and sole can be used.

1 Combine butter, 2 teaspoons lemon juice, lemon peel, mustard, tarragon and salt in small bowl; mix well with fork.

2 Spray 12-inch nonstick skillet with nonstick cooking spray; heat over medium heat. Drizzle fish with remaining 2 teaspoons lemon juice; sprinkle one side of each fillet with paprika.

3 Place fish in skillet, paprika side down; cook 3 minutes. Gently turn and cook 3 minutes longer or until fish is opaque in center and begins to flake when tested with fork. Top with butter mixture.

NUTRIENTS PER SERVING:

Calories: 170, **Total Fat:** 4g, **Saturated Fat:** 1g, **Cholesterol:** 91mg, **Sodium:** 481mg, **Carbohydrates:** 14g, **Dietary Fiber:** 4g, **Protein:** 22g
Dietary Exchange: 2½ Meat, 2 Vegetable

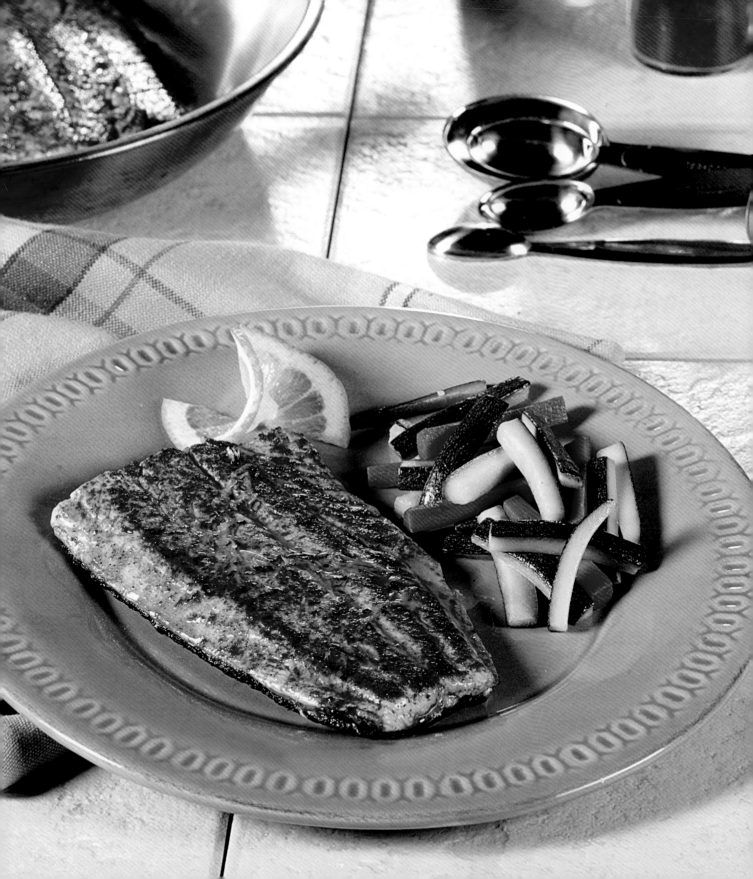

LEMON-DIJON CHICKEN WITH POTATOES

MAKES 6 SERVINGS

---

2 medium lemons

½ cup chopped fresh parsley

2 tablespoons Dijon mustard

4 cloves garlic, minced

2 teaspoons olive oil

1 teaspoon dried rosemary

¾ teaspoon black pepper

½ teaspoon salt

1 whole chicken (about 3½ pounds)

1½ pounds small red potatoes, unpeeled and halved

---

1 Preheat oven to 350°F.

2 Squeeze 3 tablespoons juice from lemons; reserve squeezed lemon halves. Combine lemon juice, parsley, mustard, garlic, oil, rosemary, pepper and salt in small bowl; mix well. Reserve 2 tablespoons mixture.

3 Place chicken on rack in shallow roasting pan. Gently slide fingers between skin and meat of chicken breasts and drumsticks to separate skin from meat, being careful not to tear skin. Spoon parsley mixture between skin and meat. (Secure breast skin with toothpicks, if necessary.) Discard any remaining parsley mixture. Place lemon halves in cavity of chicken. Bake 30 minutes.

4 Meanwhile, toss potatoes with reserved parsley mixture in medium bowl until coated. Arrange potatoes around chicken; bake 1 hour or until juices in chicken run clear and thermometer inserted into thickest part of thigh registers 165°F. Remove chicken from oven; let stand 10 minutes. Remove skin; slice chicken. Sprinkle any accumulated parsley mixture from pan over chicken and potatoes.

NUTRIENTS PER SERVING:

Calories: 294, **Total Fat:** 9g, **Saturated Fat:** 2g, **Cholesterol:** 84mg, **Sodium:** 348mg, **Carbohydrates:** 26g, **Dietary Fiber:** 3g, **Protein:** 30g
Dietary Exchange: 2 Bread/Starch, 3 Meat

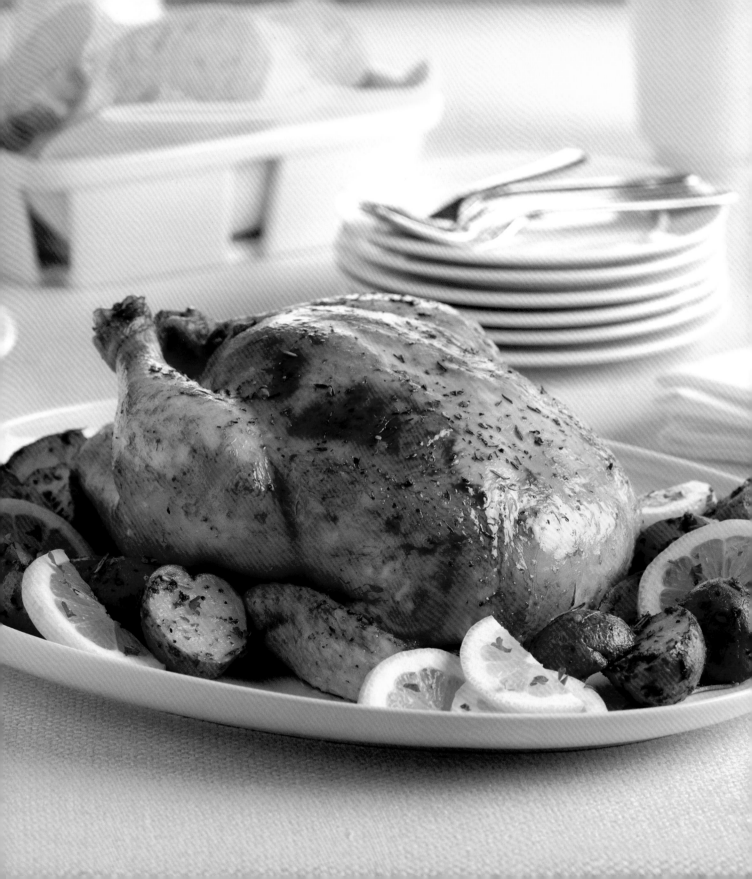

THAI-STYLE PORK KABOBS

MAKES 4 SERVINGS

⅓ cup reduced-sodium soy sauce

2 tablespoons fresh lime juice

2 tablespoons water

2 teaspoons hot chili oil*

2 cloves garlic, minced

1 teaspoon minced fresh ginger

12 ounces well-trimmed pork tenderloin

1 red and/or yellow bell pepper, cut into ½-inch pieces

1 red or sweet onion, cut into ½-inch chunks

2 cups hot cooked rice

If hot chili oil is not available, combine 2 teaspoons vegetable oil and ½ teaspoon red pepper flakes in small microwavable bowl. Microwave on HIGH 30 to 45 seconds. Let stand 5 minutes to allow flavors to develop.

1 Whisk soy sauce, lime juice, water, chili oil, garlic and ginger in medium bowl until well blended. Reserve ⅓ cup for dipping sauce.

2 Cut pork tenderloin into ½-inch strips. Add to remaining soy sauce mixture; toss to coat evenly. Cover; refrigerate at least 30 minutes or up to 2 hours, turning once.

3 Prepare grill for direct cooking. Spray grid with nonstick cooking spray.

4 Remove pork from marinade; discard marinade. Alternately thread pork strips, bell pepper and onion onto 8 (8- to 10-inch) skewers.**

5 Grill, covered, over medium heat 6 to 8 minutes or until pork is barely pink in center, turning halfway through grilling time.

6 Serve with rice and reserved dipping sauce.

***If using wooden skewers, soak in cool water 20 to 30 minutes to prevent burning.*

NUTRIENTS PER SERVING:

Calories: 248, **Total Fat:** 4g, **Saturated Fat:** 1g, **Cholesterol:** 49mg, **Sodium:** 271mg, **Carbohydrates:** 30g, **Dietary Fiber:** 2g, **Protein:** 22g
Dietary Exchange: 1½ Bread/Starch, 2 Meat, 1 Vegetable

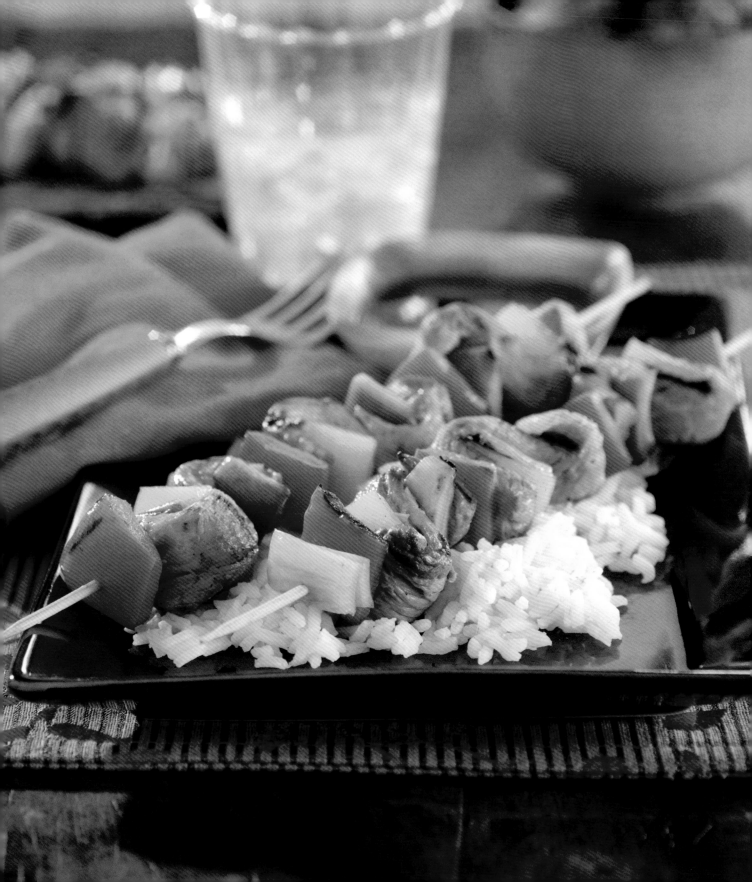

RED SNAPPER VERA CRUZ

MAKES 4 SERVINGS

---

4 **red snapper fillets (about 1 pound)**

¼ **cup fresh lime juice**

1 **tablespoon fresh lemon juice**

1 **teaspoon chili powder**

4 **green onions with 4 inches of tops, sliced into ½-inch lengths**

1 **tomato, coarsely chopped**

½ **cup chopped Anaheim or green bell pepper**

½ **cup chopped red bell pepper**

Black pepper

MICROWAVE DIRECTIONS

1 Place red snapper in shallow 9- to 10-inch round microwavable baking dish. Combine lime juice, lemon juice and chili powder in small bowl. Pour over snapper. Marinate 10 minutes, turning once or twice.

2 Sprinkle green onions, tomato, Anaheim and bell pepper over snapper. Season with black pepper. Cover dish loosely with vented plastic wrap. Microwave on HIGH 5 to 6 minutes or just until snapper flakes in center, rotating dish every 2 minutes. Let stand, covered, 4 minutes.

NOTE: Serve over hot cooked rice, if desired.

NUTRIENTS PER SERVING:

Calories: 144, **Total Fat:** 2g, **Saturated Fat:** 1g, **Cholesterol:** 42mg, **Sodium:** 61mg, **Carbohydrates:** 7g, **Dietary Fiber:** 2g, **Protein:** 24g
Dietary Exchange: 2½ Meat, 1 Vegetable

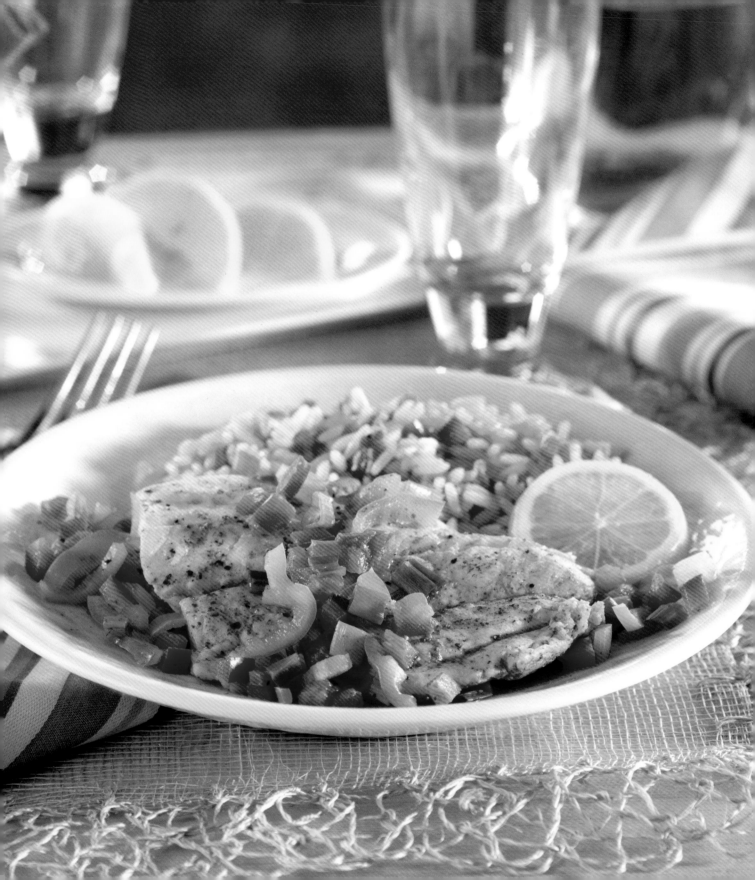

FAJITA-SEASONED GRILLED CHICKEN

MAKES 2 SERVINGS

2 boneless skinless chicken breasts (about 4 ounces each)

1 bunch green onions, ends trimmed

1 tablespoon olive oil

2 teaspoons fajita seasoning mix

1. Prepare grill for direct cooking.

2. Brush chicken and green onions with oil. Sprinkle both sides of chicken breasts with seasoning mix. Grill chicken and green onions 6 to 8 minutes or until chicken is no longer pink in center (165°F).

3. Serve chicken with green onions.

NUTRIENTS PER SERVING:

Calories: 176, **Total Fat:** 8g, **Saturated Fat:** 1g, **Cholesterol:** 43mg, **Sodium:** 186mg, **Carbohydrates:** 8g, **Dietary Fiber:** 2g, **Protein:** 19g
Dietary Exchange: 2½ Meat, 1½ Vegetable, ½ Fat

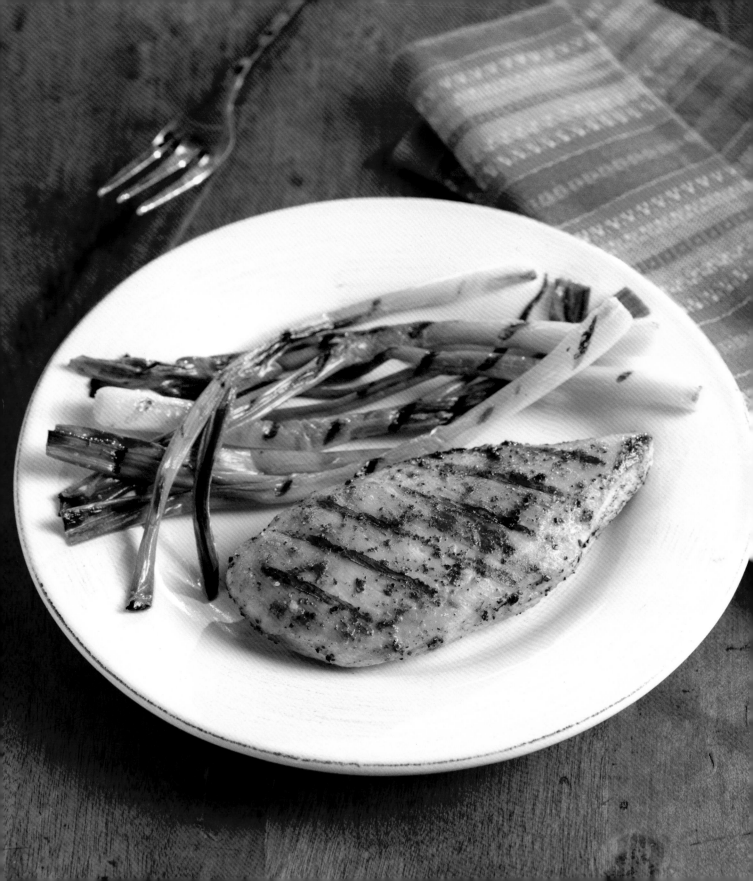

RAVIOLI WITH HOMEMADE TOMATO SAUCE

MAKES 6 SERVINGS

3 cloves garlic, peeled

½ cup fresh basil leaves

3 cups seeded peeled tomatoes, cut into quarters

2 tablespoons tomato paste

2 tablespoons prepared fat-free Italian salad dressing

1 tablespoon balsamic vinegar

¼ teaspoon black pepper

1 package (9 ounces) refrigerated reduced-fat fresh cheese ravioli

2 cups shredded washed spinach leaves

1 cup (4 ounces) shredded part-skim mozzarella cheese

MICROWAVE DIRECTIONS

1 Place garlic in food processor; process until coarsely chopped. Add basil; process until coarsely chopped. Add tomatoes, tomato paste, salad dressing, vinegar and pepper; pulse until tomatoes are chopped.

2 Spray 9-inch square microwavable dish with nonstick cooking spray. Spread 1 cup tomato sauce in dish. Layer half of ravioli and half of spinach over tomato sauce. Repeat layers with 1 cup tomato sauce and remaining ravioli and spinach; top with remaining 1 cup tomato sauce. Cover with plastic wrap; refrigerate 1 to 8 hours.

3 Vent plastic wrap. Microwave on MEDIUM (50%) 20 minutes or until pasta is tender and hot. Sprinkle with cheese. Microwave on HIGH 3 minutes or just until cheese melts. Let stand, covered, 5 minutes before serving.

NUTRIENTS PER SERVING:

Calories: 206, **Total Fat:** 6g, **Saturated Fat:** 3g, **Cholesterol:** 40mg, **Sodium:** 401mg, **Carbohydrates:** 26g, **Dietary Fiber:** 3g, **Protein:** 13g
Dietary Exchange: 1 Bread/Starch, 1 Meat, 2 Vegetable, ½ Fat

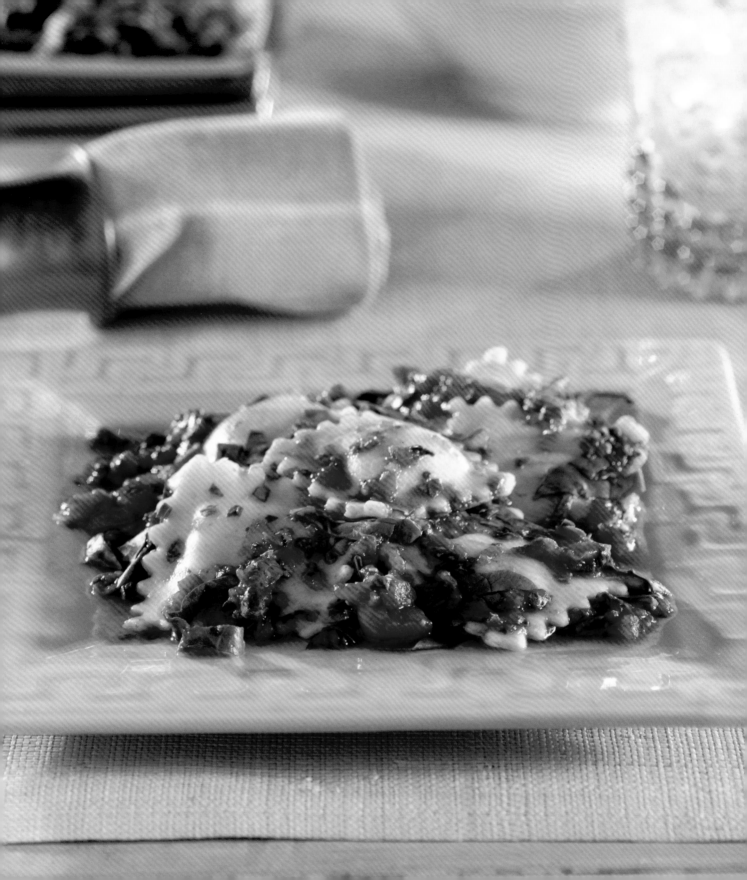

IMPOSSIBLY EASY SALMON PIE

MAKES 8 SERVINGS

1 can (7½ ounces) red salmon, drained and deboned

½ cup grated Parmesan cheese

¼ cup sliced green onions

1 jar (2 ounces) chopped pimientos, drained

½ cup low-fat (1%) cottage cheese

1 tablespoon lemon juice

1½ cups low-fat (1%) milk

¾ cup reduced-fat biscuit baking mix

2 eggs

2 egg whites *or* ¼ cup cholesterol-free egg substitute

¼ teaspoon salt

¼ teaspoon dried dill weed

¼ teaspoon paprika (optional)

1 Preheat oven to 375°F. Spray 9-inch pie plate with nonstick cooking spray.

2 Combine salmon, Parmesan cheese, green onions and pimientos in prepared pie plate.

3 Combine cottage cheese and lemon juice in blender or food processor; blend until smooth. Add milk, baking mix, eggs, egg whites, salt and dill weed; blend 15 seconds. Pour over salmon mixture in pie plate. Sprinkle with paprika, if desired.

4 Bake 35 to 40 minutes or until top is golden brown and knife inserted near center comes out clean. Let stand 5 minutes before serving.

NUTRIENTS PER SERVING:

Calories: 155, **Total Fat:** 6g, **Saturated Fat:** 2g, **Cholesterol:** 74mg, **Sodium:** 565mg, **Carbohydrates:** 11g, **Dietary Fiber:** 1g, **Protein:** 14g
Dietary Exchange: 1 Bread/Starch, 2 Meat

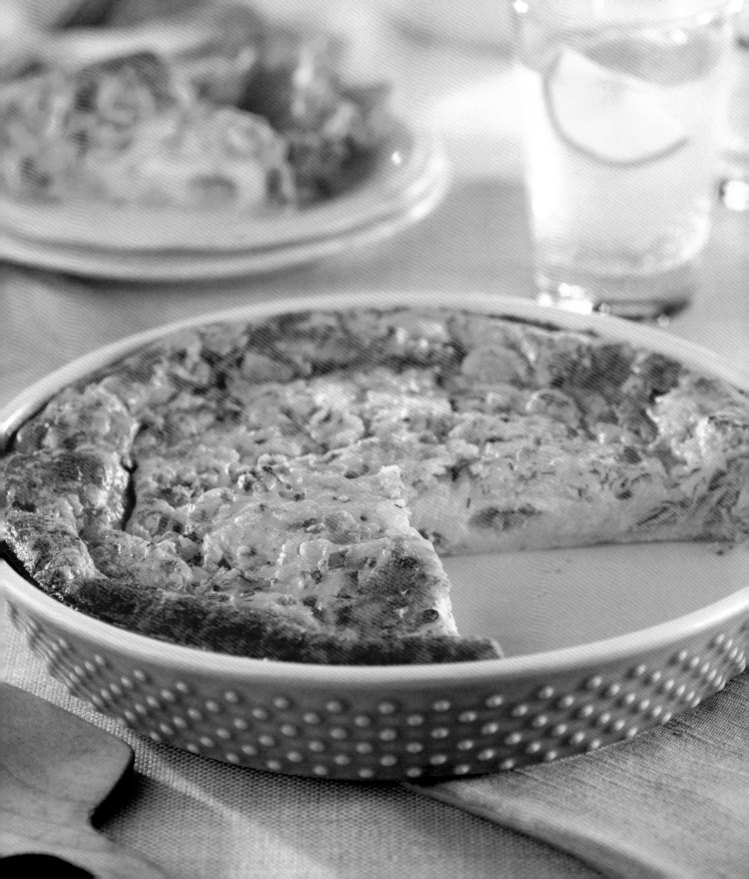

CASHEW CHICKEN

MAKES 4 SERVINGS

10 ounces boneless skinless chicken breasts, cut into 1×½-inch pieces

1 tablespoon cornstarch

1 tablespoon dry white wine

1 tablespoon reduced-sodium soy sauce

½ teaspoon garlic powder

1 teaspoon vegetable oil

6 green onions, cut into 1-inch pieces

2 cups sliced mushrooms

1 red or green bell pepper, cut into strips

1 can (6 ounces) sliced water chestnuts, rinsed and drained

2 tablespoons hoisin sauce (optional)

2 cups hot cooked rice

¼ cup cashews, toasted*

To toast cashews, spread in single layer in heavy-bottomed skillet. Cook over medium heat 1 to 2 minutes, stirring frequently, until nuts are lightly browned. Remove from skillet immediately. Cool before using.

1 Place chicken in large resealable food storage bag. Whisk cornstarch, wine, soy sauce and garlic powder in small bowl until smooth and well blended. Pour over chicken. Seal bag; turn to coat evenly. Marinate in refrigerator 1 hour.

2 Drain chicken; discard marinade. Heat oil in wok or large nonstick skillet over medium-high heat. Add green onions; cook and stir 1 minute. Add chicken; cook and stir 2 minutes or until browned. Add mushrooms, bell pepper and water chestnuts; cook and stir 3 minutes or until vegetables are crisp-tender and chicken is cooked through. Stir in hoisin sauce, if desired; cook and stir 1 minute or until heated through.

3 Serve chicken and vegetables over rice. Top with cashews.

NUTRIENTS PER SERVING:

Calories: 274, **Total Fat:** 7g, **Saturated Fat:** 1g, **Cholesterol:** 36mg, **Sodium:** 83mg, **Carbohydrates:** 34g, **Dietary Fiber:** 3g, **Protein:** 18g
Dietary Exchange: 1½ Bread/Starch, 2 Meat, 1½ Vegetable, ½ Fat

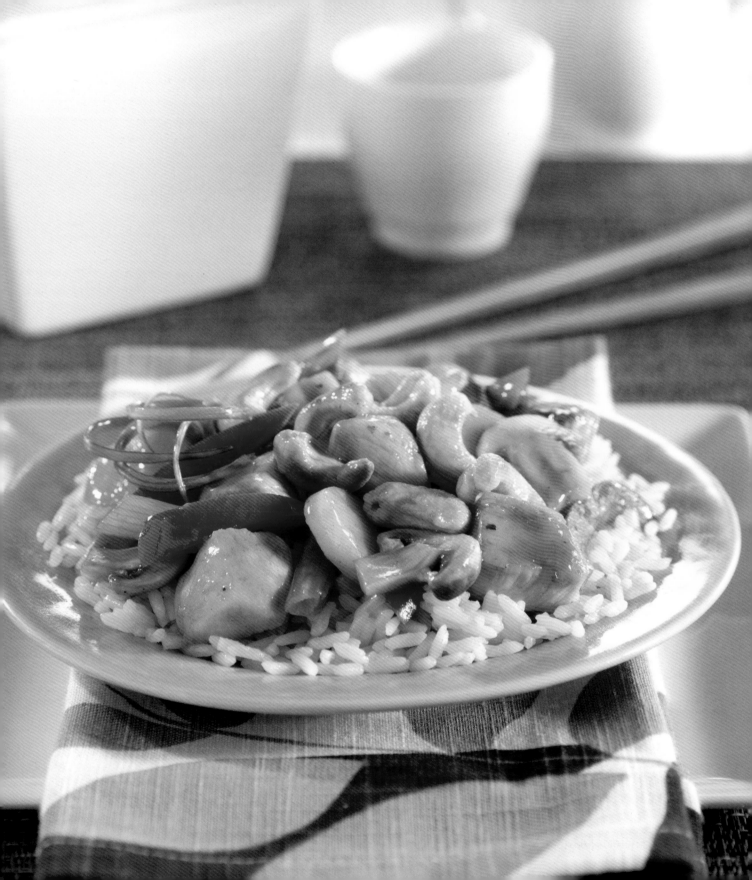

GINGER BEEF AND CARROT KABOBS

MAKES 4 SERVINGS

12 ounces boneless beef top sirloin steak (1 inch thick), cut into 1-inch cubes

¼ cup reduced-sodium soy sauce

1 tablespoon water

1 tablespoon honey

1 teaspoon olive oil

¼ teaspoon ground ginger

¼ teaspoon ground allspice

⅛ teaspoon ground red pepper

1 clove garlic, minced

2 medium carrots, cut into 1-inch pieces (1½ cups)

4 green onions, trimmed to 4-inch pieces

1 Place beef in large resealable food storage bag. Combine soy sauce, water, honey, oil, ginger, allspice, red pepper and garlic in small bowl. Pour over meat in bag. Seal bag; turn to coat meat. Marinate in refrigerator 4 to 16 hours, turning bag occasionally.

2 Meanwhile, place 1 inch water in medium saucepan. Bring water to a boil. Add carrots. Cover; cook 5 minutes or until crisp-tender. Drain.

3 Prepare grill for direct cooking. Spray grid with nonstick cooking spray. Drain meat. Discard marinade. Alternately thread meat and carrot pieces onto 4 skewers.* Add green onion piece to end of each skewer.

4 Grill kabobs over medium coals 11 to 14 minutes or until meat is tender, turning once during grilling.

*If using wooden skewers, soak in cool water 20 to 30 minutes to prevent burning.

NUTRIENTS PER SERVING:

Calories: 133, **Total Fat:** 4g, **Saturated Fat:** 1g, **Cholesterol:** 52mg, **Sodium:** 69mg, **Carbohydrates:** 5g, **Dietary Fiber:** 1g, **Protein:** 19g
Dietary Exchange: 2 Meat, 1 Vegetable

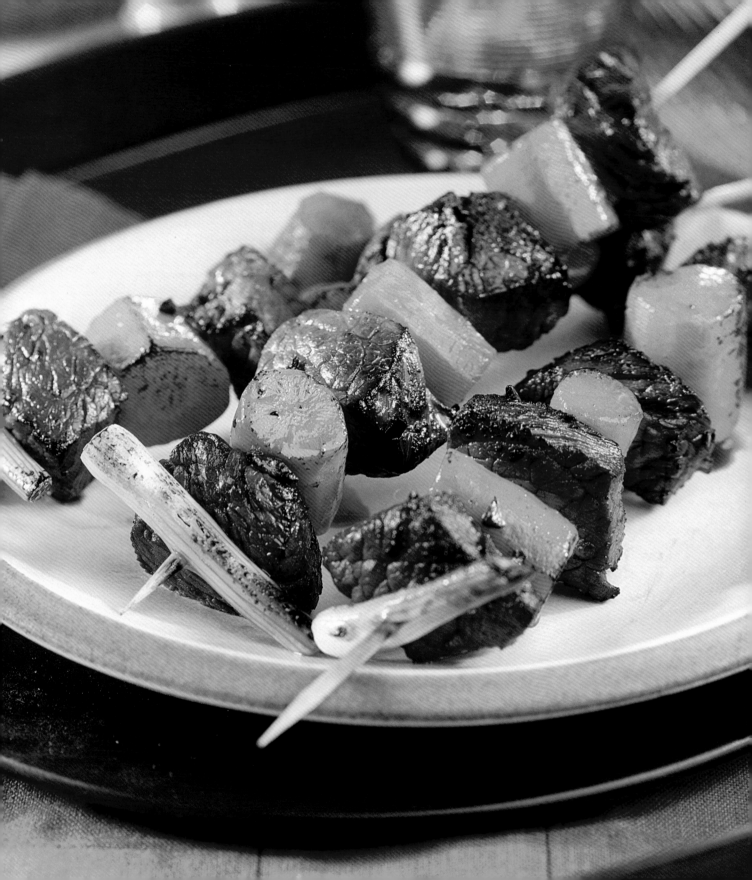

GRILLED CHICKEN ADOBO

MAKES 4 SERVINGS

½ cup chopped onion

⅓ cup lime juice

6 cloves garlic, coarsely chopped

1 teaspoon ground cumin

1 teaspoon dried oregano

½ teaspoon dried thyme

¼ teaspoon ground red pepper

4 boneless skinless chicken breasts (about 1 pound total)

3 tablespoons chopped fresh cilantro (optional)

1 Combine onion, lime juice and garlic in food processor. Process until onion is finely minced. Transfer to large resealable food storage bag. Add cumin, oregano, thyme and red pepper; knead bag until blended. Place chicken in bag; press out air and seal. Turn to coat chicken with marinade. Refrigerate 30 minutes or up to 4 hours, turning occasionally.

2 Prepare grill for direct cooking. Spray grid with nonstick cooking spray. Remove chicken from marinade; discard marinade. Place chicken on grid. Grill 5 to 7 minutes on each side over medium heat or until chicken is no longer pink in center. Transfer to clean serving platter and garnish with cilantro, if desired.

NUTRIENTS PER SERVING:

Calories: 139, **Total Fat:** 3g, **Saturated Fat:** 1g, **Cholesterol:** 69mg, **Sodium:** 61mg, **Carbohydrates:** 1g, **Dietary Fiber:** 1g, **Protein:** 25g
Dietary Exchange: 3 Meat

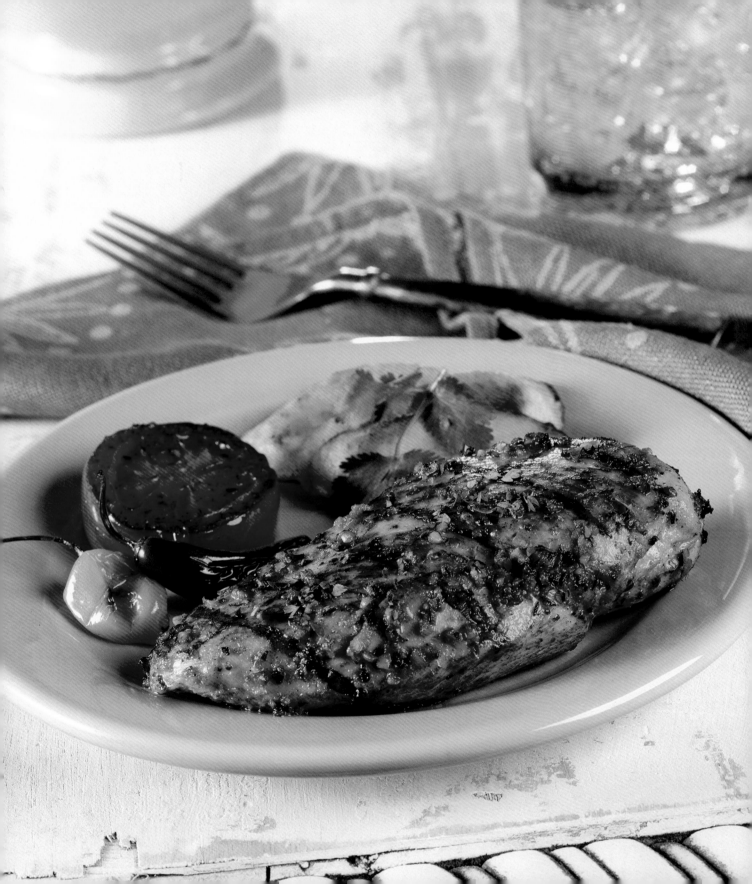

SEARED SPICED PORK TENDERLOIN AND APPLES

MAKES 4 SERVINGS

½ teaspoon ground cinnamon

½ teaspoon ground cumin

½ teaspoon black pepper

¼ teaspoon salt

⅛ teaspoon ground allspice

1 pound pork tenderloin

1 teaspoon canola oil

2 medium Fuji or Gala apples, sliced

¼ cup raisins

¼ cup water

2 teaspoons light margarine

1 Preheat oven to 425°F. Line baking sheet with foil. Combine cinnamon, cumin, pepper, salt and allspice in small bowl; mix well. Sprinkle evenly over all sides of pork, pressing to adhere.

2 Heat oil in large skillet over medium-high heat. Add pork; cook until browned on all sides, turning frequently. Transfer to prepared baking sheet.

3 Bake pork 18 minutes or until barely pink in center. Transfer to cutting board; let stand 5 minutes before cutting into thin slices.

4 Meanwhile, place apples, raisins and water in same skillet; cook and stir over medium-high heat 2 minutes or until apples begin to brown. Remove from heat; stir in margarine. Cover and let stand until ready to serve. To serve, place about ⅓ cup apple mixture on plate; top with pork slices.

NUTRIENTS PER SERVING:

Calories: 217, **Total Fat:** 6g, **Saturated Fat:** 2g, **Cholesterol:** 73mg, **Sodium:** 216mg, **Carbohydrates:** 17g, **Dietary Fiber:** 2g, **Protein:** 26g
Dietary Exchange: 3 Meat, 1 Fruit

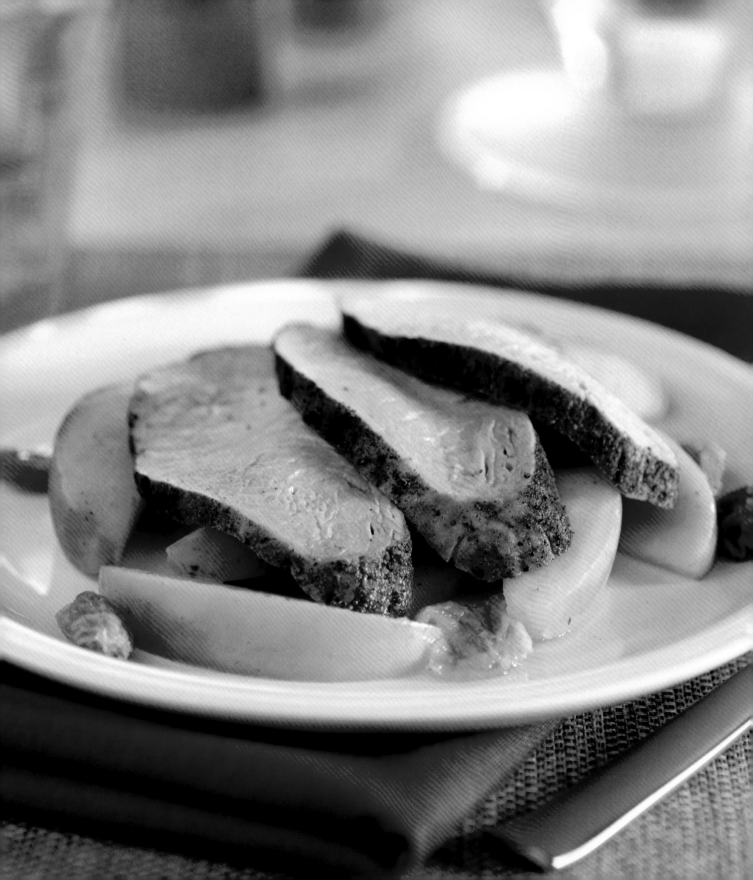

BAKED FISH WITH TOMATOES & HERBS

MAKES 4 SERVINGS

4 lean white fish fillets (about 1 pound), such as orange roughy or sole

2 tablespoons plus 2 teaspoons lemon juice, divided

½ teaspoon paprika

1 cup finely chopped seeded tomatoes

2 tablespoons capers, rinsed and drained

2 tablespoons finely chopped fresh parsley

1½ teaspoons dried basil

2 teaspoons olive oil

¼ teaspoon salt

1 Preheat oven to 350°F. Coat 12×8-inch glass baking dish with nonstick cooking spray.

2 Arrange fish fillets in dish. Drizzle 2 tablespoons lemon juice over fillets; sprinkle with paprika. Cover with foil; bake 18 minutes or until opaque in center and flakes easily when tested with fork.

3 Meanwhile, in medium saucepan, combine tomatoes, capers, parsley, remaining 2 teaspoons lemon juice, basil, oil and salt. Five minutes before fish is done, place saucepan over high heat. Bring to a boil. Reduce heat and simmer 2 minutes or until hot. Remove from heat.

4 Serve fish topped with tomato mixture.

NUTRIENTS PER SERVING:

Calories: 150, **Total Fat:** 4g, **Saturated Fat:** 1g, **Cholesterol:** 42mg, **Sodium:** 360mg, **Carbohydrates:** 4g, **Dietary Fiber:** 1g, **Protein:** 24g
Dietary Exchange: 3 Meat, 1 Vegetable

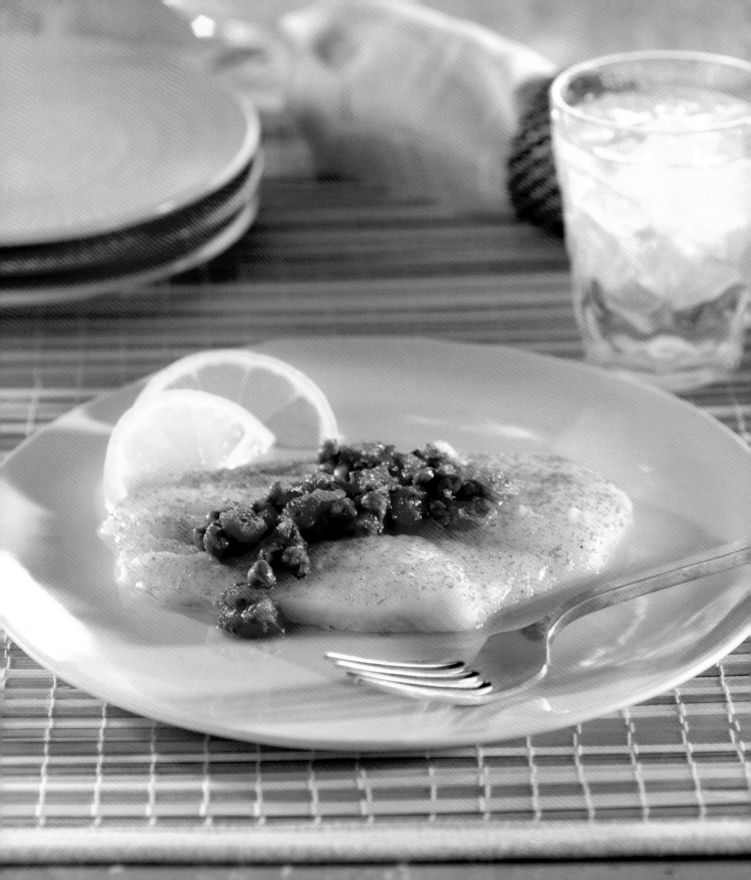

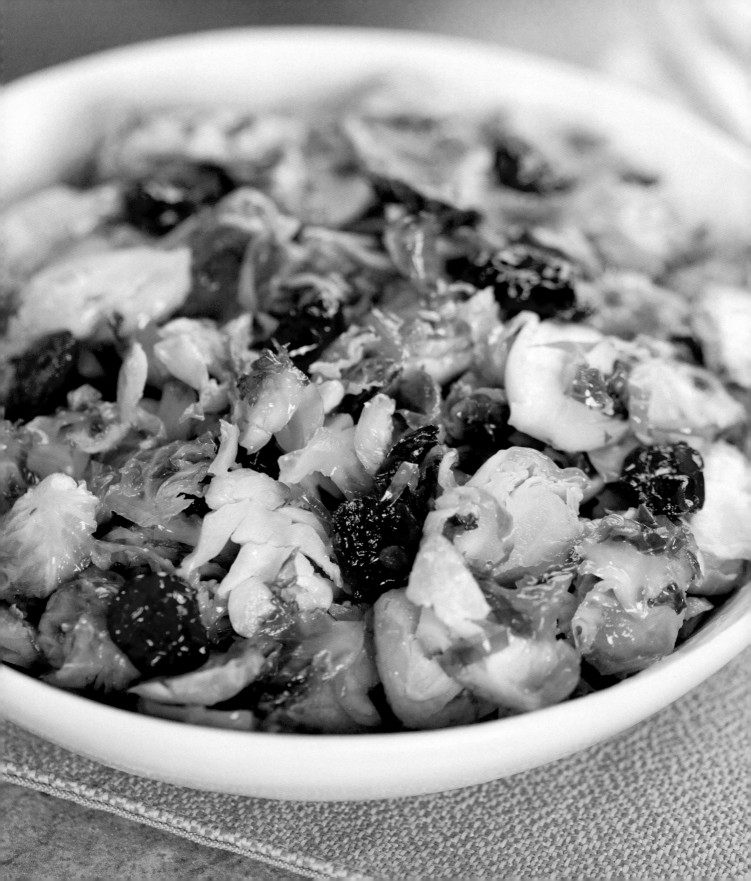

Salads & Sides

CARAMELIZED BRUSSELS SPROUTS WITH CRANBERRIES

MAKES 4 SERVINGS

---

1 tablespoon vegetable oil

1 pound Brussels sprouts, ends trimmed, thinly sliced

¼ cup dried cranberries

2 teaspoons packed brown sugar

¼ teaspoon salt

---

1 Heat oil in large skillet over medium-high heat. Add Brussels sprouts; cook 10 minutes or until crisp-tender and beginning to brown, stirring occasionally.

2 Add cranberries, brown sugar and salt; cook and stir 5 minutes or until Brussels sprouts are browned.

NUTRIENTS PER SERVING:

Calories: 105, **Total Fat:** 4g, **Saturated Fat:** 1g, **Cholesterol:** 0mg, **Sodium:** 317mg, **Carbohydrates:** 17g, **Dietary Fiber:** 4g, **Protein:** 3g
Dietary Exchange: 2 Vegetable, ½ Fruit, ½ Fat

ROASTED BEET RISOTTO

MAKES 4 SERVINGS

---

2 medium beets, trimmed

4 cups vegetable broth

1 tablespoon canola oil

1 cup uncooked arborio rice

1 leek, finely chopped

½ cup crumbled goat cheese, plus additional for garnish

1 teaspoon Italian seasoning

¼ teaspoon salt

Juice of 1 lemon

Lemon wedges (optional)

---

1 Preheat oven to 400°F. Wrap each beet tightly in foil. Place on baking sheet. Roast 45 minutes to 1 hour or until knife inserted into centers goes in easily. Unwrap beets; discard foil. Let stand 15 minutes or until cool enough to handle. Peel and cut beets into bite-size pieces. Set aside.

2 Heat broth to a simmer in medium saucepan; keep warm.

3 Heat oil in large saucepan over medium-high heat. Add rice; cook and stir 1 to 2 minutes. Add leek; cook and stir 1 to 2 minutes. Add broth, ½ cup at a time, stirring constantly until broth is absorbed before adding next ½ cup. Continue adding broth and stirring until rice is tender and mixture is creamy, about 20 to 25 minutes. Remove from heat.

4 Stir ½ cup goat cheese, Italian seasoning and salt into risotto. Gently stir in beets. Sprinkle with lemon juice and additional cheese, if desired. Garnish with lemon wedges. Serve immediately.

NUTRIENTS PER SERVING:

Calories: 278, **Total Fat:** 8g, **Saturated Fat:** 3g, **Cholesterol:** 9mg, **Sodium:** 383mg, **Carbohydrates:** 45g, **Dietary Fiber:** 2g, **Protein:** 8g
Dietary Exchange: 3 Bread/Starch, 2 Fat

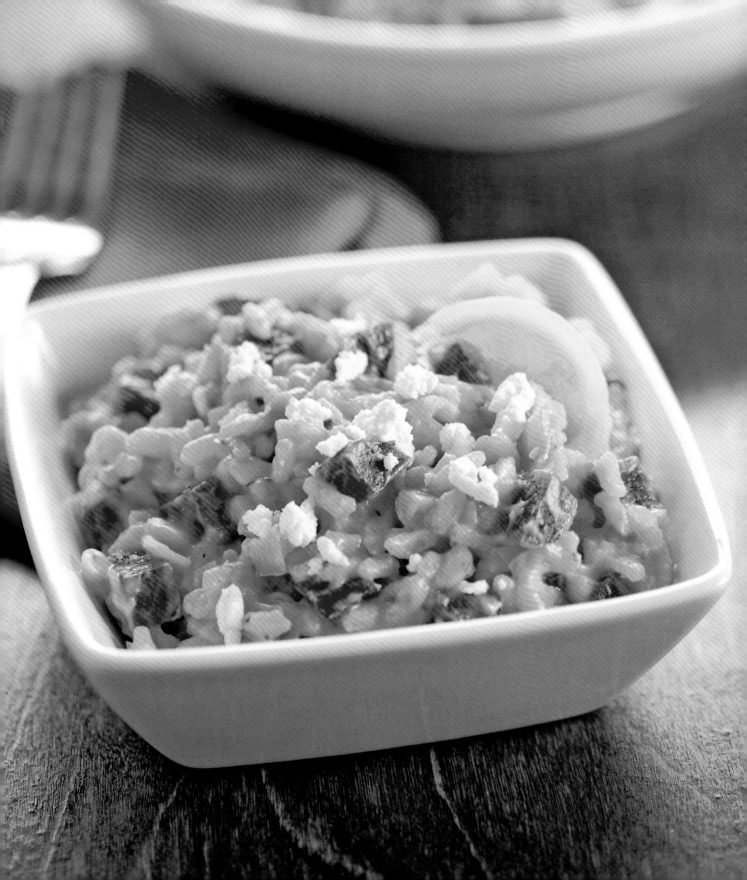

HEIRLOOM TOMATO QUINOA SALAD

MAKES 4 SERVINGS

---

1 cup uncooked quinoa

2 cups water

2 tablespoons olive oil

1 tablespoon lemon juice

1 clove garlic, minced

½ teaspoon salt

2 cups assorted heirloom grape tomatoes (red, yellow or a combination), halved

¼ cup crumbled fat-free feta cheese

¼ cup chopped fresh basil, plus additional basil leaves for garnish

---

1 Place quinoa in fine-mesh strainer; rinse well under cold running water. Bring 2 cups water to a boil in small saucepan; stir in quinoa. Reduce heat to low; cover and simmer 10 to 15 minutes or until quinoa is tender and water is absorbed.

2 Meanwhile, whisk oil, lemon juice, garlic and salt in large bowl until well blended. Gently stir in tomatoes and quinoa. Cover; refrigerate at least 30 minutes.

3 Stir in feta cheese just before serving. Top each serving with 1 tablespoon chopped basil. Garnish with additional basil leaves.

NUTRIENTS PER SERVING:

Calories: 246, **Total Fat:** 10g, **Saturated Fat:** 1g, **Cholesterol:** 1mg, **Sodium:** 387mg, **Carbohydrates:** 32g, **Dietary Fiber:** 4g, **Protein:** 9g
Dietary Exchange: 2 Bread/Starch, 1 Meat, 1 Fat

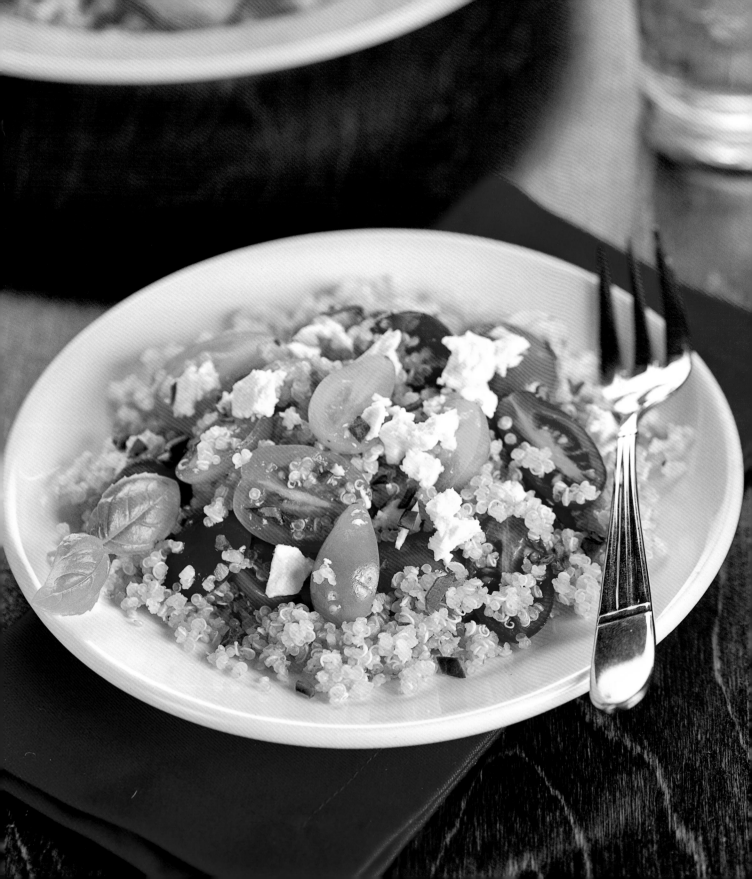

GRILLED STONE FRUIT SALAD

MAKES 4 SERVINGS

2 tablespoons fresh orange juice

1 tablespoon fresh lemon juice

2 teaspoons canola oil

1 teaspoon honey

½ teaspoon Dijon mustard

1 tablespoon finely chopped fresh mint

1 medium peach, halved and pit removed

1 medium nectarine, halved and pit removed

1 medium plum, halved and pit removed

4 cups mixed baby greens

½ cup crumbled goat cheese

1. Prepare grill for direct cooking over medium-high heat. Spray grid with nonstick cooking spray.

2. Whisk orange juice, lemon juice, oil, honey and mustard in small bowl until smooth and well blended. Stir in mint.

3. Brush cut sides of fruits with orange juice mixture. Set remaining dressing aside. Place fruits, cut sides down, on prepared grid. Grill, covered, 2 to 3 minutes. Turn over; grill 2 to 3 minutes or until fruits begin to soften. Remove to plate; let stand to cool slightly. When cool enough to handle, cut into wedges.

4. Arrange mixed greens on 4 serving plates. Top evenly with fruits and goat cheese. Drizzle with remaining dressing. Serve immediately.

NUTRIENTS PER SERVING:

Calories: 119, **Total Fat:** 6g, **Saturated Fat:** 3g, **Cholesterol:** 11mg, **Sodium:** 91mg, **Carbohydrates:** 14g, **Dietary Fiber:** 2g, **Protein:** 4g
Dietary Exchange: 1 Fruit, 1 Fat

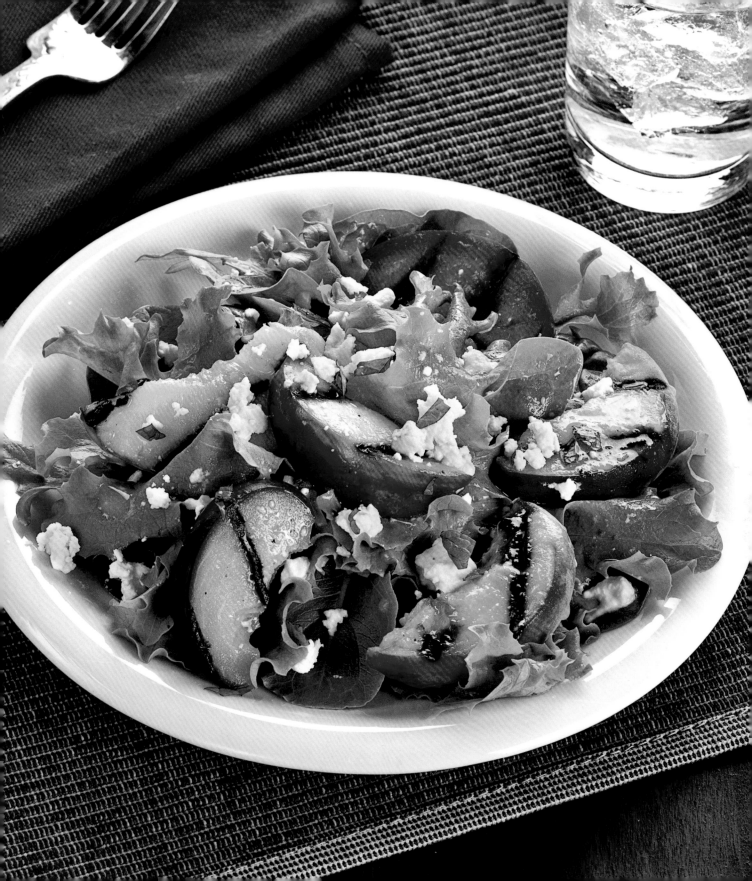

COLD PEANUT NOODLE AND EDAMAME SALAD

MAKES 4 SERVINGS

½ of an 8-ounce package brown rice pad thai noodles

3 tablespoons soy sauce

2 tablespoons dark sesame oil

2 tablespoons unseasoned rice vinegar

1 tablespoon sugar

1 tablespoon finely grated fresh ginger

1 tablespoon creamy peanut butter

1 tablespoon sriracha or hot chili sauce

2 teaspoons minced garlic

½ cup thawed frozen shelled edamame

¼ cup shredded carrots

¼ cup sliced green onions

Chopped peanuts (optional)

1 Prepare noodles according to package directions for pasta. Rinse under cold water; drain. Cut noodles into 3-inch lengths. Place in large bowl; set aside.

2 Whisk soy sauce, oil, vinegar, sugar, ginger, peanut butter, sriracha and garlic in small bowl until smooth and well blended.

3 Pour dressing over noodles; toss gently to coat. Stir in edamame and carrots. Cover and refrigerate at least 30 minutes before serving. Top with green onions and peanuts, if desired.

NOTE: Brown rice pad thai noodles can be found in the Asian section of the supermarket. Regular thin rice noodles or whole wheat spaghetti may be substituted.

NUTRIENTS PER SERVING:

Calories: 239, **Total Fat:** 10g, **Saturated Fat:** 1g, **Cholesterol:** 0mg, **Sodium:** 556mg, **Carbohydrates:** 32g, **Dietary Fiber:** 1g, **Protein:** 6g
Dietary Exchange: 1½ Bread/Starch, 1 Vegetable, 2 Fat

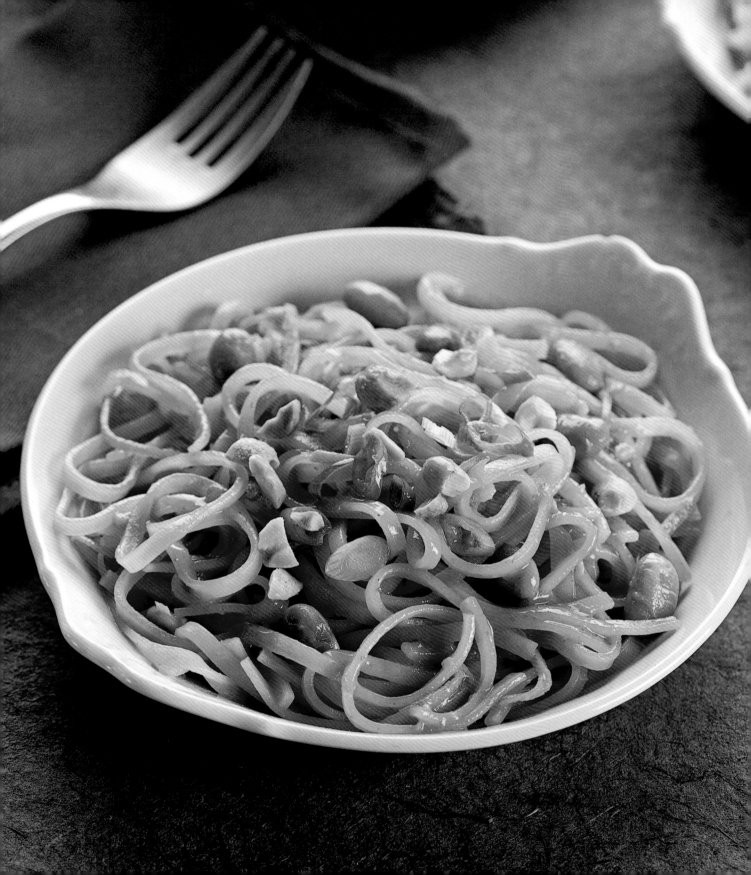

ARUGULA SALAD WITH SUN-DRIED TOMATO VINAIGRETTE

MAKES 4 SERVINGS

¼ cup sun-dried tomatoes (not packed in oil)

2 tablespoons olive oil

1 tablespoon balsamic vinegar

¼ teaspoon salt

¼ teaspoon black pepper

1 package (5 ounces) baby arugula

1 cup halved grape tomatoes

¼ cup shaved Parmesan cheese

¼ cup pine nuts, toasted* (optional)

*To toast pine nuts, spread in single layer in heavy skillet. Cook over medium heat 1 to 2 minutes or until nuts are lightly browned, stirring frequently.

---

1 Combine sun-dried tomatoes, oil, vinegar, salt and pepper in blender or food processor; blend until smooth.

2 Combine arugula and grape tomatoes in large bowl. Add dressing; toss to coat. Top with cheese and pine nuts, if desired.

NUTRIENTS PER SERVING:

Calories: 114, **Total Fat:** 9g, **Saturated Fat:** 2g, **Cholesterol:** 6mg, **Sodium:** 274mg, **Carbohydrates:** 6g, **Dietary Fiber:** 1g, **Protein:** 4g
Dietary Exchange: 1 Vegetable, 2 Fat

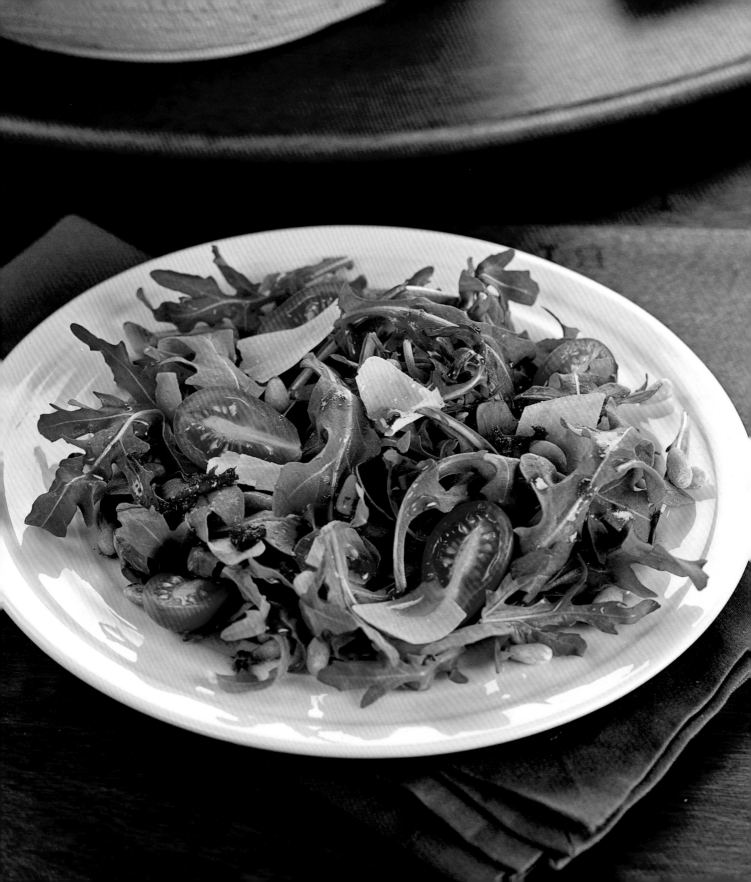

QUINOA & ROASTED VEGETABLES

MAKES 6 SERVINGS

- 2 medium sweet potatoes, cut into ½-inch-thick slices
- 1 medium eggplant, peeled and cut into ½-inch cubes
- 1 medium tomato, cut into wedges
- 1 large green bell pepper, sliced
- 1 small onion, cut into wedges
- ½ teaspoon salt
- ¼ teaspoon black pepper
- ¼ teaspoon ground red pepper
- 1 cup uncooked quinoa
- 2 cloves garlic, minced
- ½ teaspoon dried thyme
- ¼ teaspoon dried marjoram
- 2 cups water or fat-free reduced-sodium vegetable broth

1 Preheat oven to 450°F. Line large jelly-roll pan with foil; spray with nonstick cooking spray.

2 Combine sweet potatoes, eggplant, tomato, bell pepper and onion on prepared pan; spray lightly with cooking spray. Sprinkle with salt, black pepper and ground red pepper; toss to coat. Spread vegetables in single layer. Roast 20 to 30 minutes or until vegetables are browned and tender.

3 Meanwhile, place quinoa in fine-mesh strainer; rinse well under cold running water. Spray medium saucepan with cooking spray; heat over medium heat. Add garlic, thyme and marjoram; cook and stir 1 to 2 minutes. Add quinoa; cook and stir 2 to 3 minutes. Stir in 2 cups water; bring to a boil over high heat. Reduce heat to low. Simmer, covered, 15 to 20 minutes or until water is absorbed. (Quinoa will appear somewhat translucent.) Transfer quinoa to large bowl; gently stir in roasted vegetables.

NUTRIENTS PER SERVING:

Calories: 193, **Total Fat:** 2g, **Saturated Fat:** 1g, **Cholesterol:** 0mg, **Sodium:** 194mg, **Carbohydrates:** 40g, **Dietary Fiber:** 6g, **Protein:** 6g
Dietary Exchange: 2½ Bread/Starch, ½ Vegetable

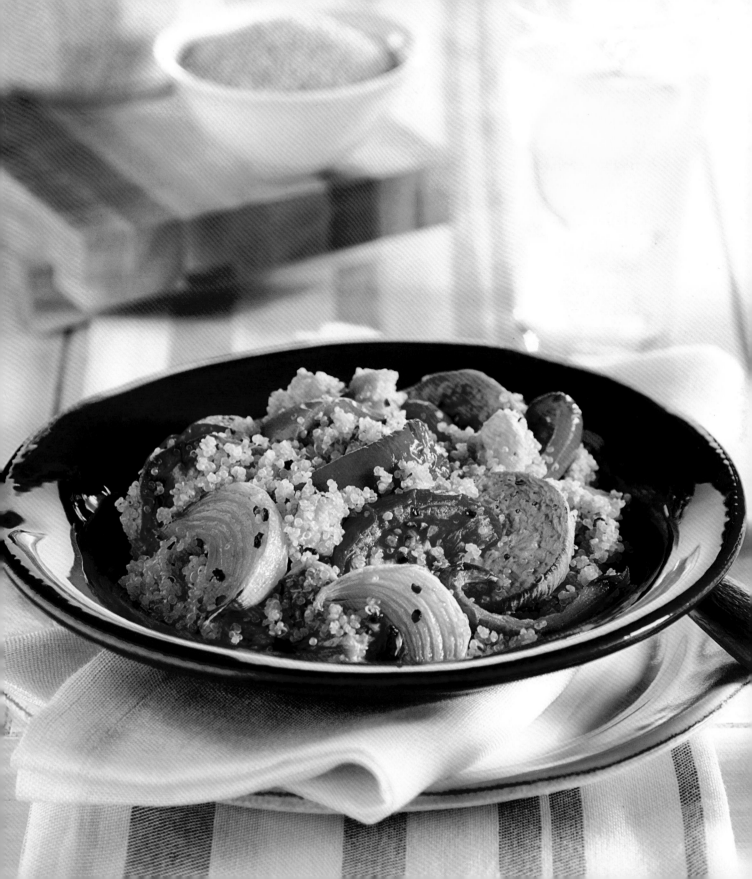

OLD-FASHIONED HERB STUFFING

MAKES 4 SERVINGS

6 slices (8 ounces) whole wheat, rye or white bread (or combination), cut into ½-inch cubes

1 tablespoon margarine or butter

1 cup chopped onion

½ cup thinly sliced celery

½ cup thinly sliced carrot

1 cup fat-free reduced-sodium chicken broth

1 tablespoon chopped fresh thyme *or* 1 teaspoon dried thyme

1 tablespoon chopped fresh sage *or* 1 teaspoon dried sage

½ teaspoon paprika

¼ teaspoon black pepper

1 Preheat oven to 350°F. Spray 1½-quart baking dish with nonstick cooking spray.

2 Place bread cubes on baking sheet; bake 10 minutes or until dry.

3 Melt margarine in large saucepan over medium heat. Add onion, celery and carrot; cook and stir 10 minutes or until vegetables are tender. Add broth, thyme, sage, paprika and pepper; bring to a simmer. Stir in bread cubes. Spoon into prepared baking dish.

4 Cover and bake 25 to 30 minutes or until heated through.

NUTRIENTS PER SERVING:

Calories: 199, **Total Fat:** 5g, **Saturated Fat:** 1g, **Cholesterol:** 0mg, **Sodium:** 395mg, **Carbohydrates:** 32g, **Dietary Fiber:** 5g, **Protein:** 8g
Dietary Exchange: 2 Bread/Starch, 1 Fat

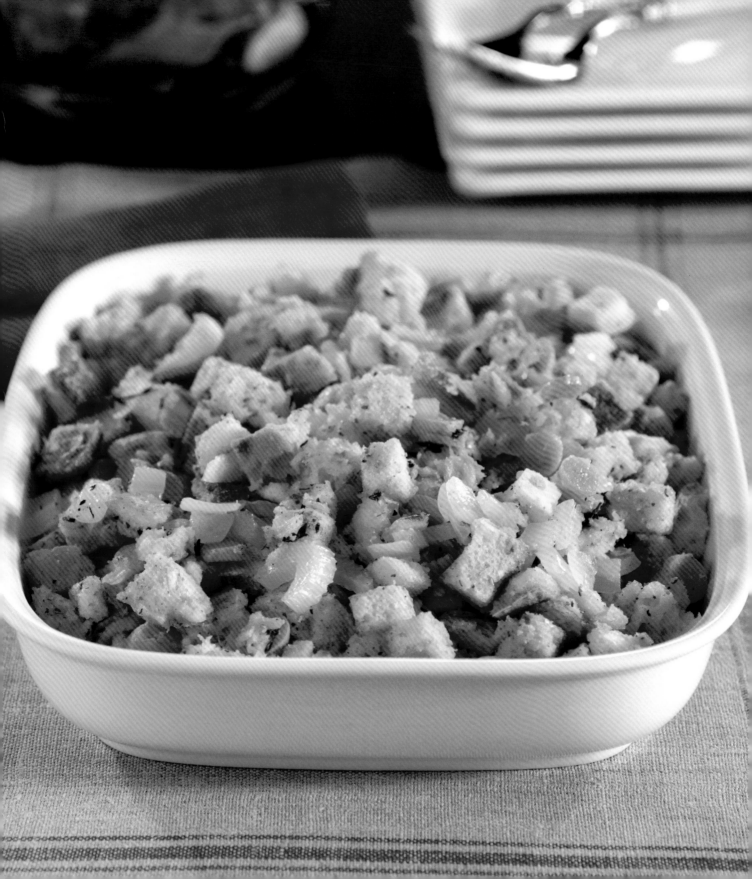

WILD RICE, MUSHROOM AND SPINACH SKILLET

MAKES 10 SERVINGS

⅓ **cup uncooked wild rice**

⅓ **cup uncooked brown rice**

⅓ **cup uncooked long grain white rice**

1½ **cups water**

1 **can (10 ounces) condensed reduced-sodium chicken broth, undiluted**

2 **tablespoons margarine**

2 **cups sliced shiitake mushrooms**

2 **cups quartered cremini (brown) mushrooms**

2 **cups sliced bok choy**

2 **cups shredded spinach leaves**

¼ **cup (1 ounce) crumbled feta cheese**

---

1 Combine wild rice, brown rice, white rice, water and broth in large saucepan. Bring to a boil over high heat. Reduce heat to low; cover and simmer 45 minutes or until rice is tender.

2 Melt margarine in large skillet over medium heat. Add mushrooms; cook and stir 3 minutes. Add bok choy and spinach; cook and stir 3 minutes or until greens are wilted.

3 Add rice to greens in skillet; stir until blended. Sprinkle with feta cheese just before serving.

NUTRIENTS PER SERVING:

Calories: 130, **Total Fat:** 4g, **Saturated Fat:** 2g, **Cholesterol:** 6mg, **Sodium:** 117mg, **Carbohydrates:** 19g, **Dietary Fiber:** 2g, **Protein:** 4g
Dietary Exchange: 1 Bread/Starch, 1 Vegetable, ½ Fat

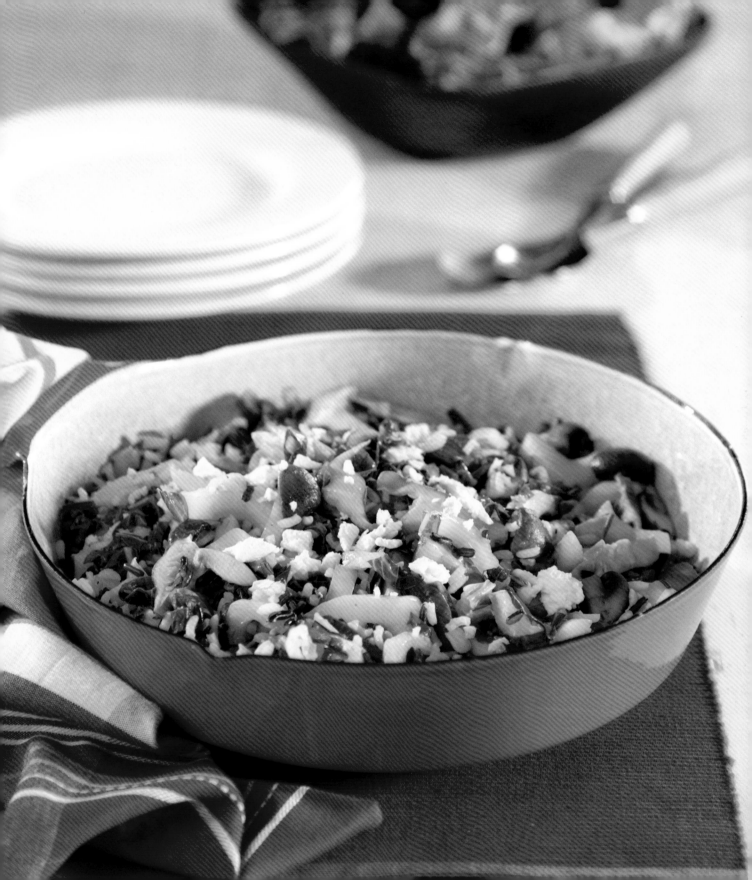

CONFETTI BLACK BEANS

MAKES 6 SERVINGS

---

1 cup dried black beans

3 cups water

1 can (about 14 ounces) reduced-sodium chicken broth

1 bay leaf

1½ teaspoons olive oil

1 medium onion, chopped

¼ cup chopped red bell pepper

¼ cup chopped yellow bell pepper

2 cloves garlic, minced

1 jalapeño pepper, finely chopped

1 large tomato, seeded and chopped

½ teaspoon salt

⅛ teaspoon black pepper

Hot pepper sauce (optional)

---

1 Sort and rinse beans; cover with water. Soak 8 hours or overnight. Drain.

2 Combine beans and broth in large saucepan; bring to a boil over high heat. Add bay leaf. Reduce heat to low. Cover; simmer 1½ hours or until beans are tender.

3 Heat oil in large nonstick skillet over medium heat. Add onion, bell peppers, garlic and jalapeño pepper; cook and stir 8 to 10 minutes or until onion is translucent. Add tomato, salt and black pepper; cook 5 minutes.

4 Add onion mixture to beans; cook 15 to 20 minutes.

5 Remove and discard bay leaf. Serve with hot pepper sauce, if desired.

NUTRIENTS PER SERVING:

Calories: 146, **Total Fat:** 2g, **Saturated Fat:** 1g, **Cholesterol:** 0mg, **Sodium:** 209mg, **Carbohydrates:** 24g, **Dietary Fiber:** 6g, **Protein:** 8g
Dietary Exchange: 1½ Bread/Starch, ½ Meat, ½ Fat

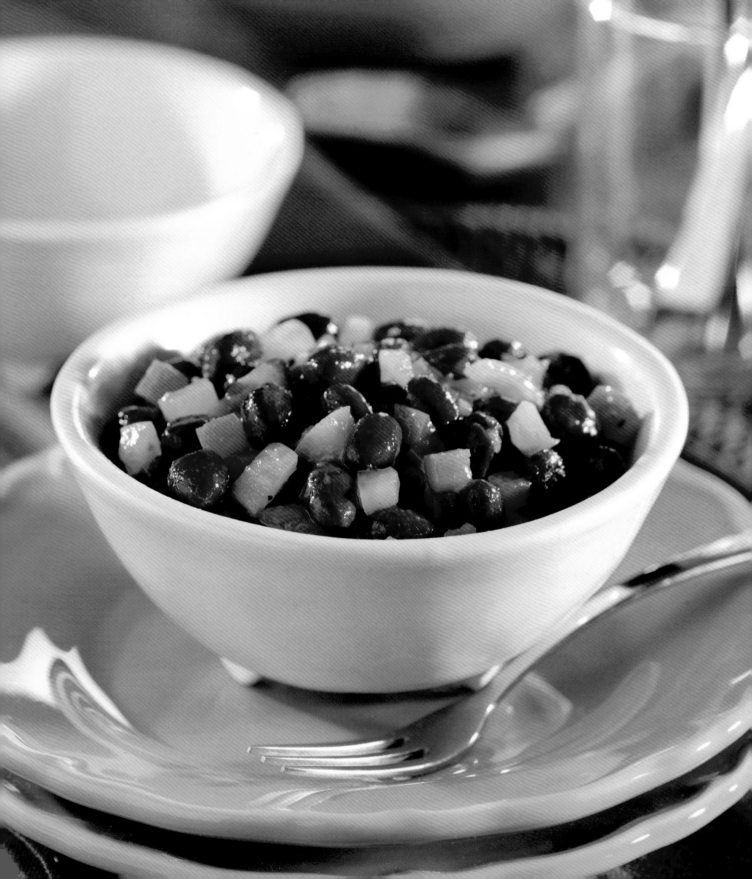

GREEN BEAN RICE WITH ALMONDS

MAKES 6 SERVINGS

2 tablespoons light margarine

½ cup finely chopped onion

1¼ cups fat-free reduced-sodium chicken broth

½ teaspoon lemon-pepper seasoning

1 cup diagonally sliced green beans

1¼ cups uncooked instant white rice

3 tablespoons sliced almonds, toasted*

To toast almonds, spread in single layer in heavy skillet. Cook over medium heat 1 to 2 minutes or until nuts are lightly browned, stirring frequently.

1 Melt margarine in medium saucepan over medium heat; add onion. Cook and stir 5 minutes or until onion is tender. Add broth and lemon-pepper seasoning; bring to a boil over high heat. Add beans; cover. Reduce heat to low; simmer 7 minutes or until beans are tender, stirring occasionally.

2 Stir rice into saucepan; cover. Remove from heat. Let stand 5 minutes or until liquid is absorbed and rice is tender. Fluff rice mixture with fork; stir in almonds until well blended. Serve immediately.

NUTRIENTS PER SERVING:

Calories: 128, **Total Fat:** 4g, **Saturated Fat:** 1g, **Cholesterol:** 0mg, **Sodium:** 53mg, **Carbohydrates:** 20g, **Dietary Fiber:** 1g, **Protein:** 3g
Dietary Exchange: 1 Bread/Starch, 1 Vegetable, ½ Fat

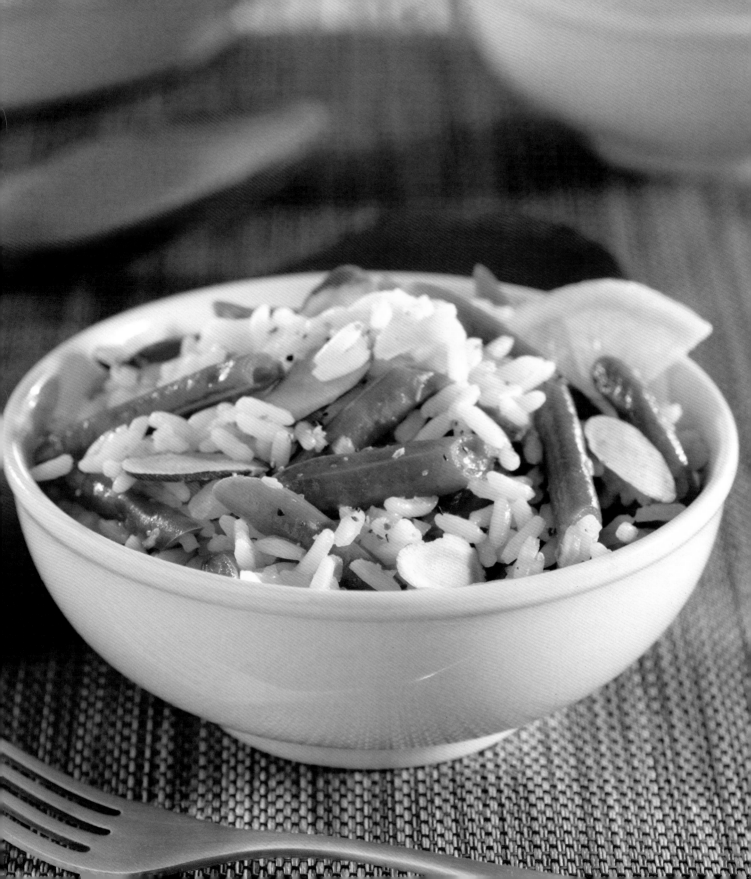

LEMON BROCCOLI PASTA

MAKES 6 SERVINGS

3 tablespoons sliced green onions

1 clove garlic, minced

2 cups fat-free reduced-sodium chicken broth

1½ teaspoons grated lemon peel

⅛ teaspoon black pepper

2 cups fresh or frozen broccoli florets

3 ounces uncooked angel hair pasta

⅓ cup reduced-fat sour cream

2 tablespoons grated reduced-fat Parmesan cheese

1 Generously spray large nonstick saucepan with nonstick cooking spray; heat over medium heat until hot. Add green onions and garlic; cook and stir 3 minutes or until onions are tender.

2 Stir broth, lemon peel and pepper into saucepan; bring to a boil over high heat. Stir in broccoli and pasta; return to a boil. Reduce heat to low. Simmer, uncovered, 6 to 7 minutes or until pasta is tender, stirring frequently.

3 Remove saucepan from heat. Stir in sour cream until well blended. Let stand 5 minutes. Top with Parmesan cheese before serving. Garnish as desired.

NUTRIENTS PER SERVING:

Calories: 100, **Total Fat:** 2g, **Saturated Fat:** 1g, **Cholesterol:** 6mg, **Sodium:** 176mg, **Carbohydrates:** 14g, **Dietary Fiber:** 3g, **Protein:** 7g
Dietary Exchange: ½ Bread/Starch, 1½ Vegetable, ½ Fat

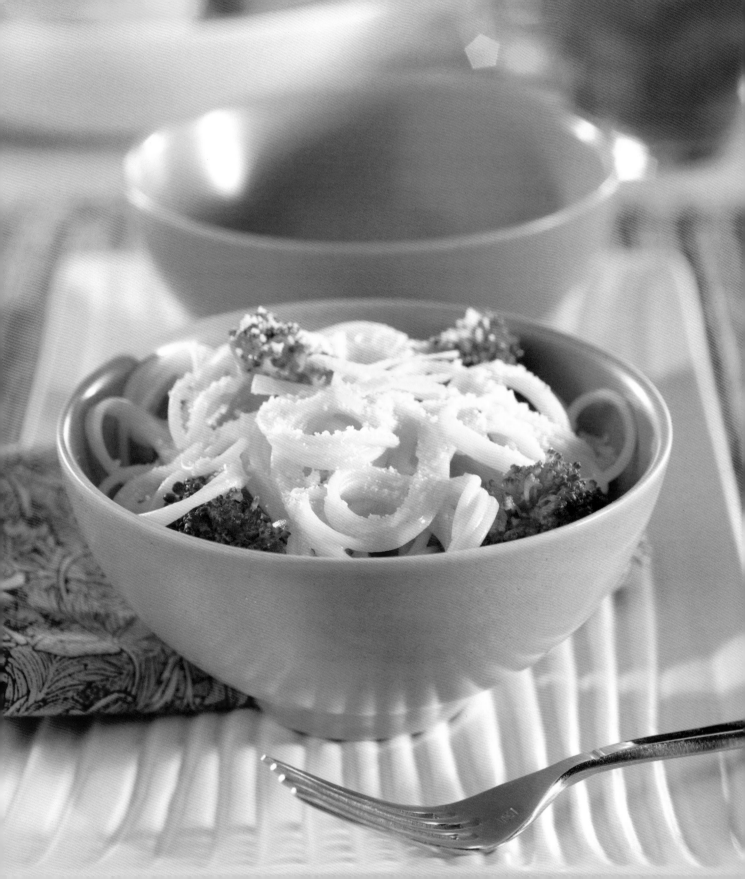

POTATO-CAULIFLOWER MASH

MAKES 4 SERVINGS

3 cups water

2 cups cubed unpeeled Yukon Gold potatoes (about 12 ounces)

10 ounces frozen cauliflower florets

¼ cup fat-free evaporated milk

2 tablespoons light margarine

¾ teaspoon salt

¼ teaspoon black pepper

1 Bring water to a boil in large saucepan. Add potatoes and cauliflower; return to a boil. Reduce heat; cover and simmer 10 minutes or until potatoes are tender.

2 Drain vegetables; place in blender with evaporated milk, margarine, salt and pepper. Blend until smooth, scraping side frequently.

NUTRIENTS PER SERVING:

Calories: 173, **Total Fat:** 6g, **Saturated Fat:** 1g, **Cholesterol:** 0mg, **Sodium:** 531mg, **Carbohydrates:** 25g, **Dietary Fiber:** 3g, **Protein:** 4g
Dietary Exchange: 1 Bread/Starch, 2 Vegetable, 1 Fat

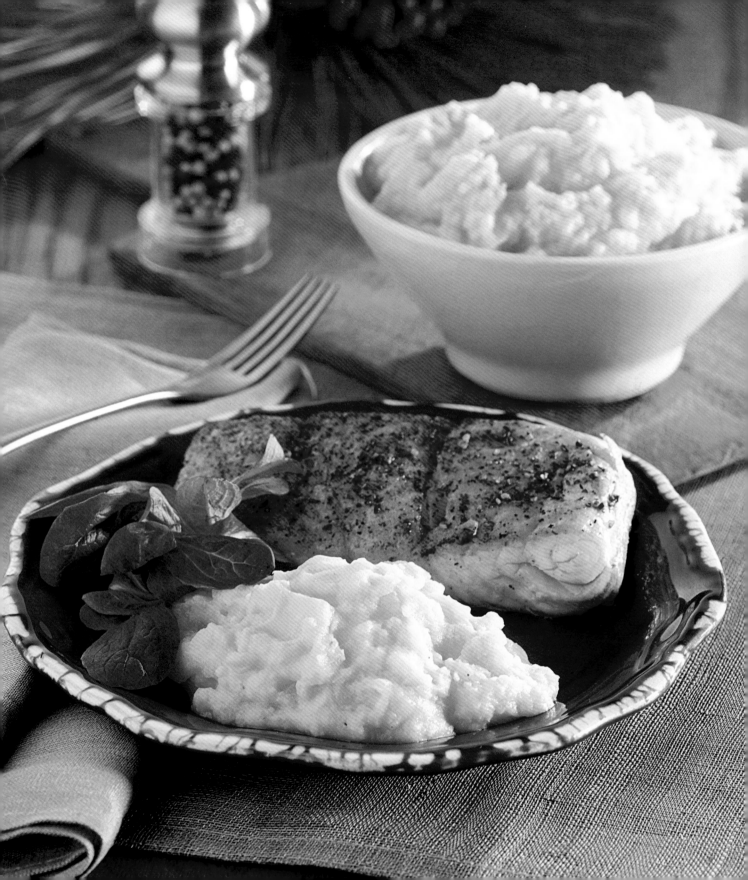

CHARRED CORN SALAD

MAKES 6 SERVINGS

---

3 tablespoons fresh lime juice

½ teaspoon salt

¼ cup extra virgin olive oil

4 to 6 ears corn, husked (enough to make 3 to 4 cups kernels)

⅔ cup canned black beans, rinsed and drained

½ cup chopped fresh cilantro

2 teaspoons minced seeded chipotle pepper (about 1 canned chipotle pepper in adobo sauce)*

Chipotle peppers in adobo sauce are available canned in the Mexican food section of most supermarkets. Since only a small amount is needed for this dish, spoon leftovers into a covered food storage container and refrigerate or freeze.

---

1 Whisk lime juice and salt in small bowl. Gradually whisk in oil until well blended. Set aside.

2 Cut corn kernels off cobs. Heat large skillet over medium-high heat. Cook corn in single layer 15 to 17 minutes or until browned and tender, stirring frequently. Transfer to large bowl to cool slightly.

3 Place beans in small microwavable bowl; microwave on HIGH 1 minute or until heated through. Add beans, cilantro and chipotle pepper to corn; mix well. Pour lime juice mixture over corn mixture; stir gently to coat.

NUTRIENTS PER SERVING:

Calories: 217, **Total Fat:** 10g, **Saturated Fat:** 1g, **Cholesterol:** 0mg, **Sodium:** 301mg, **Carbohydrates:** 29g, **Dietary Fiber:** 3g, **Protein:** 5g
Dietary Exchange: 2 Bread/Starch, 2 Fat

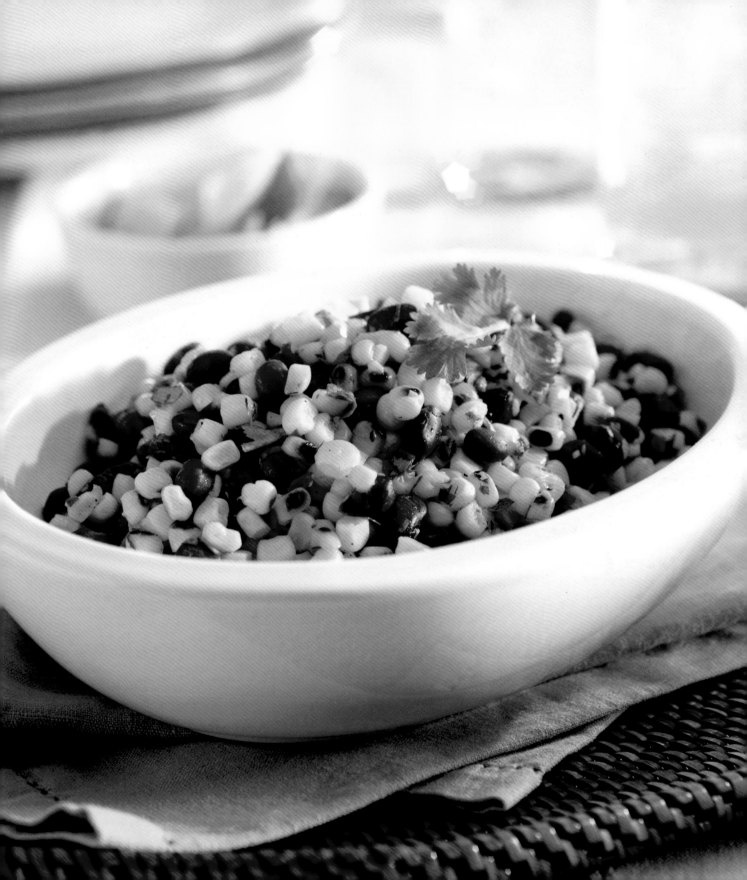

SPINACH SALAD WITH POMEGRANATE VINAIGRETTE

MAKES 4 SERVINGS

1 package (5 ounces) baby spinach

½ cup pomegranate seeds (arils)

¼ cup crumbled goat cheese

2 tablespoons chopped walnuts, toasted*

¼ cup pomegranate juice

2 tablespoons olive oil

1 tablespoon red wine vinegar

1 tablespoon honey

¼ teaspoon salt

¼ teaspoon black pepper

To toast walnuts, spread in single layer in heavy-bottomed skillet. Cook over medium heat 1 to 2 minutes, stirring frequently, until nuts are lightly browned. Remove from skillet immediately. Cool before using.

1 Combine spinach, pomegranate seeds, goat cheese and walnuts in large bowl.

2 Whisk pomegranate juice, oil, vinegar, honey, salt and pepper in small bowl until well blended. Pour over salad; gently toss to coat. Serve immediately.

TIP: For easier removal of pomegranate seeds, cut a pomegranate into pieces and immerse in a bowl of cold water. The membrane that holds the seeds in place will float to the top; discard it and collect the seeds. For convenience, you can find containers of ready-to-use pomegranate seeds in the refrigerated produce section of some supermarkets.

NUTRIENTS PER SERVING:

Calories: 161, **Total Fat:** 11g, **Saturated Fat:** 3g, **Cholesterol:** 4mg, **Sodium:** 210mg, **Carbohydrates:** 12g, **Dietary Fiber:** 1g, **Protein:** 4g
Dietary Exchange: 2 Vegetable, 2½ Fat

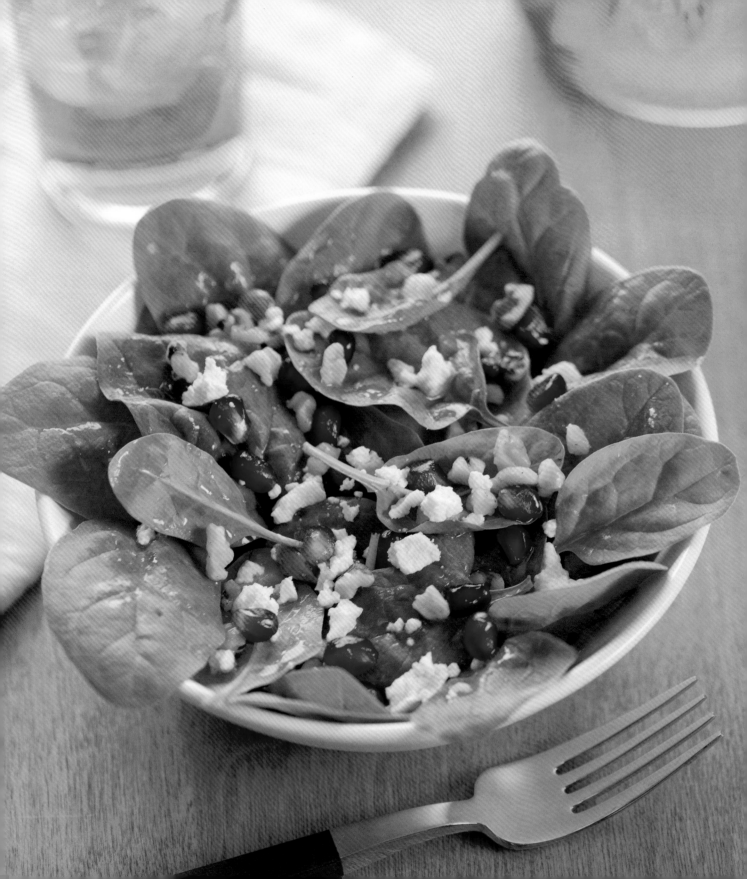

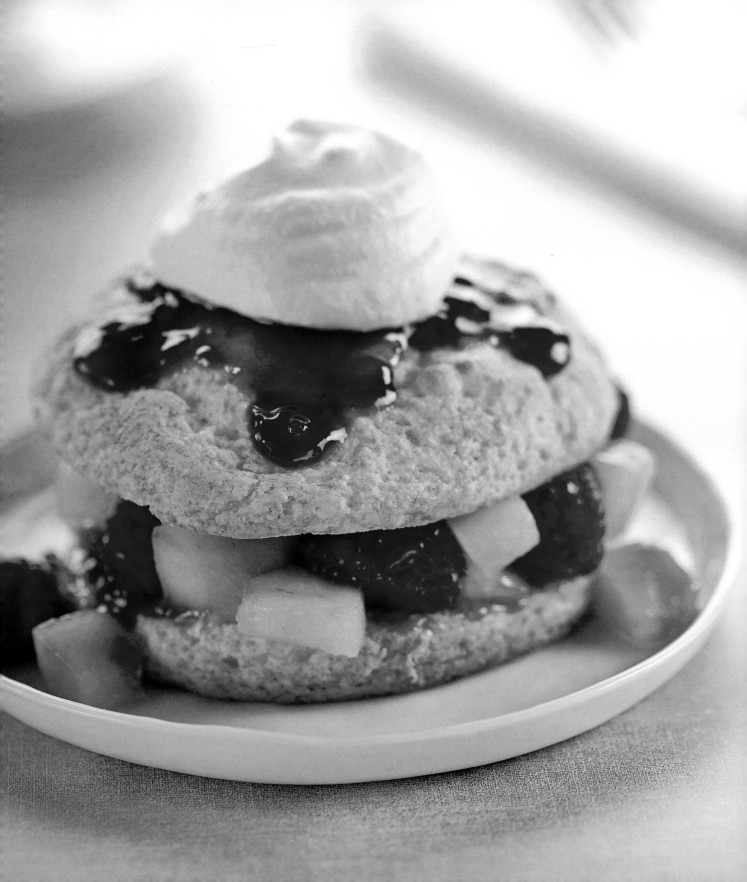

Touch of Sweetness

PEACH-MELBA SHORTCAKES

MAKES 4 SERVINGS

---

1 cup reduced-fat biscuit baking mix

¼ cup fat-free (skim) milk

2 tablespoons sugar

1¼ cups fresh raspberries

1 cup diced peeled peaches

2 tablespoons raspberry fruit spread

4 tablespoons thawed frozen whipped topping

---

1. Preheat oven to 425°F. Stir baking mix, milk and sugar in small bowl until smooth and well blended. Drop about 3 tablespoons per biscuit onto ungreased baking sheet. Bake 10 to 12 minutes or until tops are slightly browned. Cool on baking sheet 5 minutes.

2. Meanwhile, combine raspberries and peaches in medium bowl; set aside.

3. Microwave fruit spread in small microwavable bowl on HIGH 15 seconds or until softened.

4. Slice warm biscuits in half. Arrange biscuit bottoms on 4 serving plates. Drizzle ½ teaspoon fruit spread over each biscuit bottom. Top evenly with raspberries and peaches. Replace biscuit tops. Drizzle each shortcake with 1 teaspoon fruit spread; top with 1 tablespoon whipped topping.

NUTRIENTS PER SERVING:

Calories: 205, **Total Fat:** 3g, **Saturated Fat:** 1g, **Cholesterol:** 0mg, **Sodium:** 335mg, **Carbohydrates:** 42g, **Dietary Fiber:** 4g, **Protein:** 4g
Dietary Exchange: 2 Bread/Starch, 1 Fruit

CINNAMON PEAR CRISP

MAKES 12 SERVINGS

8 pears, peeled and sliced

¾ cup unsweetened apple juice concentrate

½ cup golden raisins

¼ cup plus 3 tablespoons all-purpose flour, divided

1 teaspoon ground cinnamon

⅓ cup quick oats

3 tablespoons packed dark brown sugar

3 tablespoons margarine, melted

1 Preheat oven to 375°F. Spray 11×7-inch baking dish with nonstick cooking spray.

2 Combine pears, apple juice concentrate, raisins, 3 tablespoons flour and cinnamon in large bowl; mix well. Transfer to prepared baking dish.

3 Combine oats, remaining ¼ cup flour, brown sugar and margarine in medium bowl; stir until mixture resembles coarse crumbs. Sprinkle evenly over pear mixture.

4 Bake 1 hour or until topping is golden brown.

NUTRIENTS PER SERVING:

Calories: 179, **Total Fat:** 4g, **Saturated Fat:** 1g, **Cholesterol:** 0mg, **Sodium:** 40mg, **Carbohydrates:** 38g, **Dietary Fiber:** 3g, **Protein:** 2g
Dietary Exchange: ½ Bread/Starch, 2 Fruit, ½ Fat

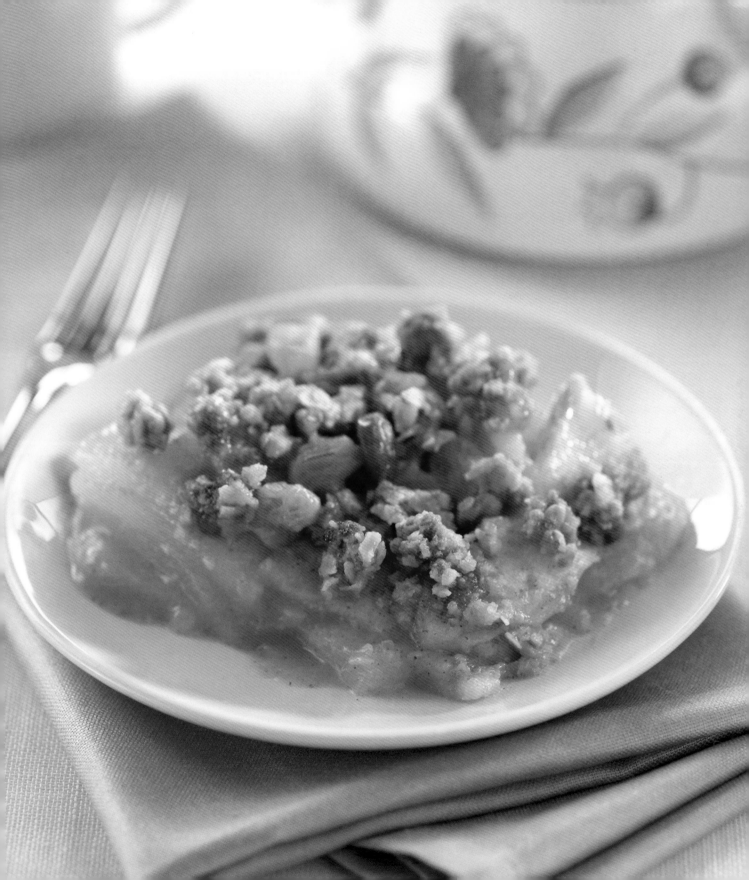

NEW-FASHIONED GINGERBREAD CAKE

MAKES 9 SERVINGS

- 2 cups cake flour
- 1 teaspoon baking powder
- 1 teaspoon ground ginger
- ½ teaspoon baking soda
- ½ teaspoon ground cinnamon
- ½ teaspoon ground nutmeg
- ¼ teaspoon ground cloves
- ¾ cup water
- ⅓ cup packed brown sugar
- ¼ cup molasses
- 3 tablespoons canola oil
- 2 tablespoons finely minced crystallized ginger (optional)
- 2 tablespoons powdered sugar

1. Preheat oven to 350°F. Spray 8-inch square baking pan with nonstick cooking spray.

2. Combine flour, baking powder, ground ginger, baking soda, cinnamon, nutmeg and cloves in large bowl; mix well. Beat water, brown sugar, molasses and oil in small bowl with electric mixer at low speed until well blended. Pour into flour mixture; beat just until blended. Stir in crystallized ginger, if desired. Pour into prepared pan.

3. Bake 30 to 35 minutes or until toothpick inserted into center comes out clean. Let cool 10 minutes. Sprinkle with powdered sugar just before serving.

NUTRIENTS PER SERVING:

Calories: 188, **Total Fat:** 5g, **Saturated Fat:** 1g, **Cholesterol:** 0mg, **Sodium:** 133mg, **Carbohydrates:** 34g, **Dietary Fiber:** 1g, **Protein:** 2g
Dietary Exchange: 2 Bread/Starch, 1 Fat

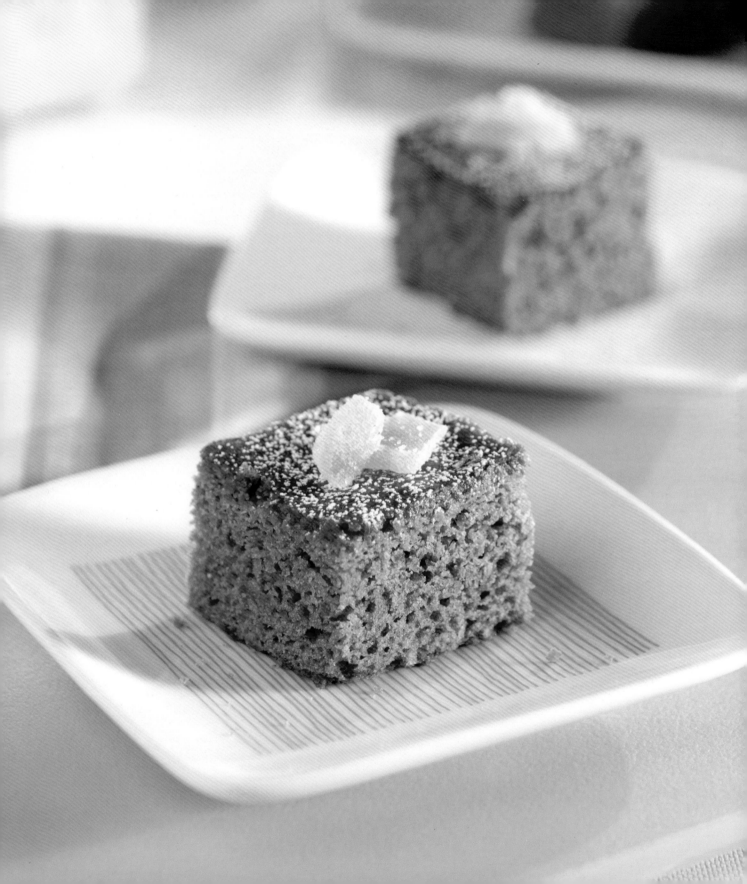

CRANBERRY-ORANGE BREAD PUDDING

MAKES 9 SERVINGS

- 2 cups (4 slices) cubed cinnamon bread
- ¼ cup dried cranberries
- 2 cups low-fat (1%) milk
- ½ cup cholesterol-free egg substitute
- 1 package (4-serving size) vanilla fat-free sugar-free pudding and pie filling mix*

- 1 teaspoon grated orange peel
- 1 teaspoon vanilla
- ½ teaspoon ground cinnamon

Do not use instant pudding and pie filling mix.

1. Preheat oven to 325°F. Spray 9 (4-ounce) custard cups with nonstick cooking spray.

2. Divide bread cubes evenly among custard cups; bake 10 minutes. Sprinkle evenly with cranberries.

3. Combine remaining ingredients in medium bowl. Pour into custard cups over cranberries. Let stand 5 to 10 minutes.

4. Bake 25 to 30 minutes or until centers are almost set. Let stand 10 minutes before serving.

NUTRIENTS PER SERVING:

Calories: 67, **Total Fat:** 1g, **Saturated Fat:** 1g, **Cholesterol:** 2mg, **Sodium:** 190mg, **Carbohydrates:** 11g, **Dietary Fiber:** 1g, **Protein:** 4g
Dietary Exchange: 1 Bread/Starch

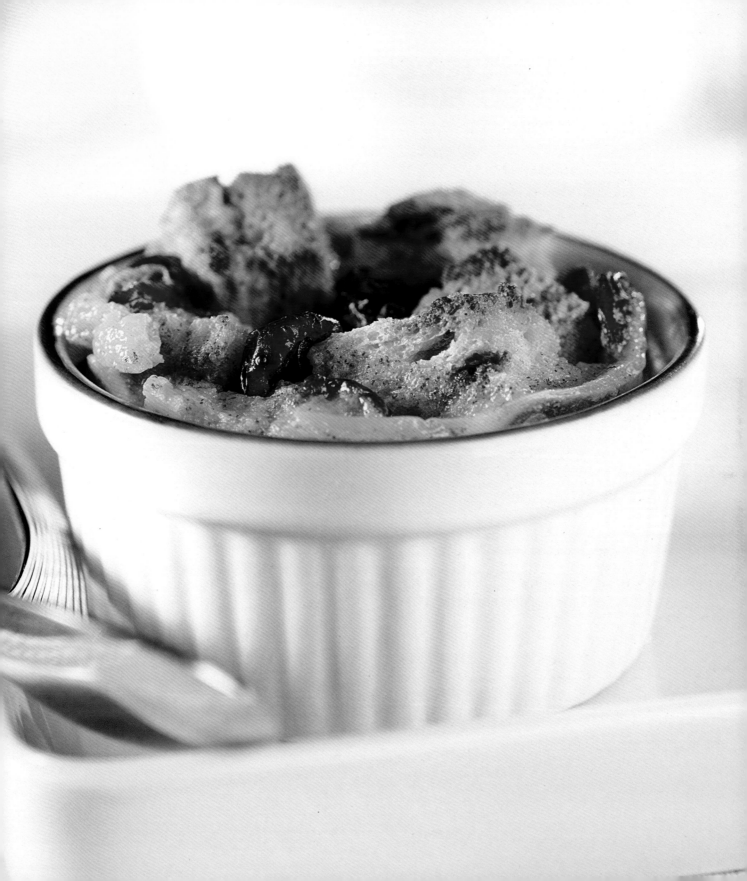

PEANUT BUTTER & BANANA COOKIES

MAKES 2 DOZEN COOKIES

¼ **cup (½ stick) butter**

½ **cup mashed ripe banana**

½ **cup no-sugar-added natural peanut butter**

¼ **cup frozen unsweetened apple juice concentrate, thawed**

1 **egg**

1 **teaspoon vanilla**

1 **cup all-purpose flour**

½ **teaspoon baking soda**

¼ **teaspoon salt**

½ **cup chopped salted peanuts**

Whole salted peanuts (optional)

1 Preheat oven to 375°F. Grease cookie sheets or lightly coat with nonstick cooking spray.

2 Beat butter in large bowl until creamy. Add banana and peanut butter; beat until smooth. Blend in apple juice concentrate, egg and vanilla. Beat in flour, baking soda and salt. Stir in chopped peanuts.

3 Drop dough by rounded tablespoonfuls 2 inches apart onto prepared cookie sheets; top each with 1 whole peanut, if desired.

4 Bake 8 minutes or until set. Cool completely on wire racks. Store in tightly covered container.

NUTRIENTS PER SERVING:

Calories: 100, **Total Fat:** 6g, **Saturated Fat:** 2g, **Cholesterol:** 14mg, **Sodium:** 88mg, **Carbohydrates:** 9g, **Dietary Fiber:** 1g, **Protein:** 3g
Dietary Exchange: ½ Bread/Starch, 1½ Fat

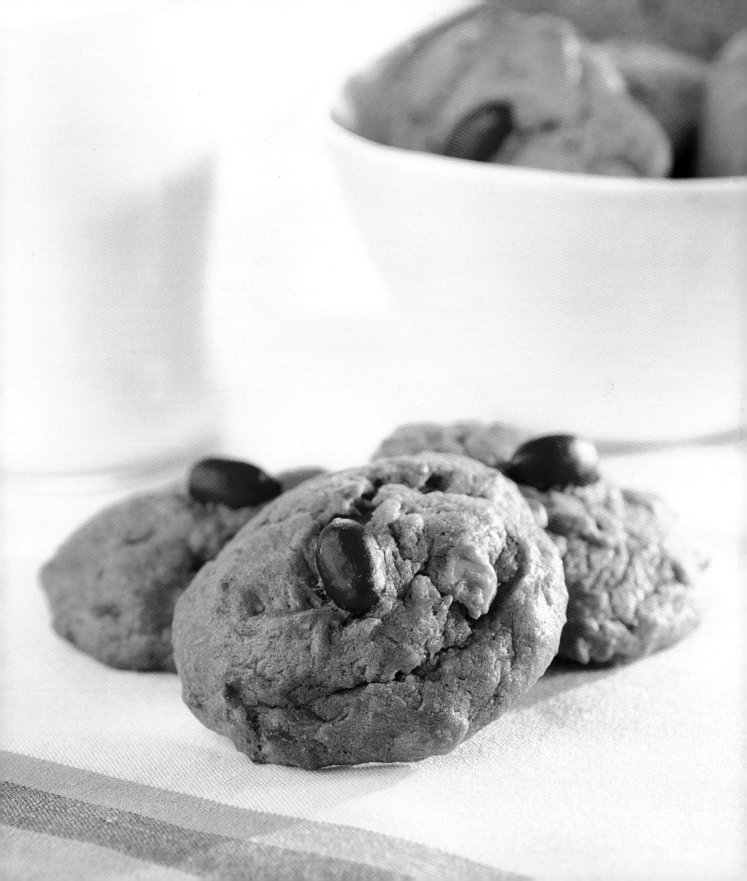

MICROWAVE CHOCOLATE PUDDING

MAKES 4 SERVINGS

¼ **cup unsweetened cocoa powder**

2 **tablespoons cornstarch**

1½ **cups reduced-fat (2%) milk**

6 **to 8 packets sugar substitute or equivalent of ⅓ cup sugar**

1 **teaspoon vanilla**

⅛ **teaspoon ground cinnamon**

Assorted sprinkles (optional)

MICROWAVE DIRECTIONS

1 Combine cocoa and cornstarch in medium microwavable bowl or 1-quart glass measure. Gradually whisk in milk until well blended.

2 Microwave on HIGH 2 minutes; stir. Microwave on MEDIUM-HIGH (70%) 3½ to 4½ minutes or until thickened, stirring every 1½ minutes.

3 Stir in sugar substitute, vanilla and cinnamon. Let stand at least 5 minutes before serving, stirring occasionally to prevent skin from forming. Serve warm or chilled. Garnish with sprinkles just before serving.

NUTRIENTS PER SERVING:

Calories: 139, **Total Fat:** 2g, **Saturated Fat:** 1g, **Cholesterol:** 7mg, **Sodium:** 50mg, **Carbohydrates:** 28g, **Dietary Fiber:** 1g, **Protein:** 4g
Dietary Exchange: 1 Bread/Starch, ½ Milk, ½ Fat

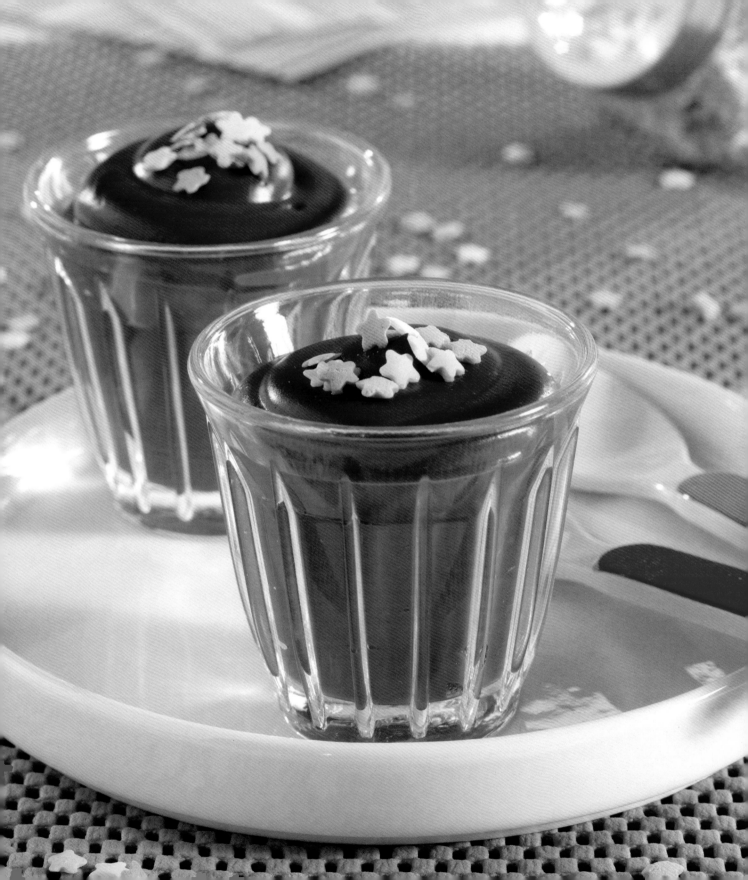

GINGERBREAD SQUARES

MAKES 9 SQUARES

---

3 tablespoons butter, softened

2 tablespoons packed light brown sugar

¼ cup molasses

1 egg white

1¼ cups all-purpose flour

½ teaspoon baking soda

½ teaspoon ground ginger

½ teaspoon ground cinnamon

¼ teaspoon salt

1 cup sweetened applesauce

Decorations: tube frostings, colored sugars, red hot cinnamon candies or other small candies (optional)

---

1 Preheat oven to 350°F. Spray 8-inch square baking pan with nonstick cooking spray; set aside.

2 Beat butter and brown sugar in medium bowl until well blended. Beat in molasses and egg white.

3 Combine dry ingredients in small bowl; mix well. Add to butter mixture alternately with applesauce, mixing well after each addition. Transfer batter to prepared pan.

4 Bake 25 to 30 minutes or until toothpick inserted into center comes out clean. Cool completely on wire rack. Cut into 9 squares. Frost and decorate, if desired.

NUTRIENTS PER SERVING:

Calories: 151, **Total Fat:** 4g, **Saturated Fat:** 2g, **Cholesterol:** 11mg, **Sodium:** 175mg, **Carbohydrates:** 26g, **Dietary Fiber:** 1g, **Protein:** 2g
Dietary Exchange: 1½ Bread/Starch, 1 Fat

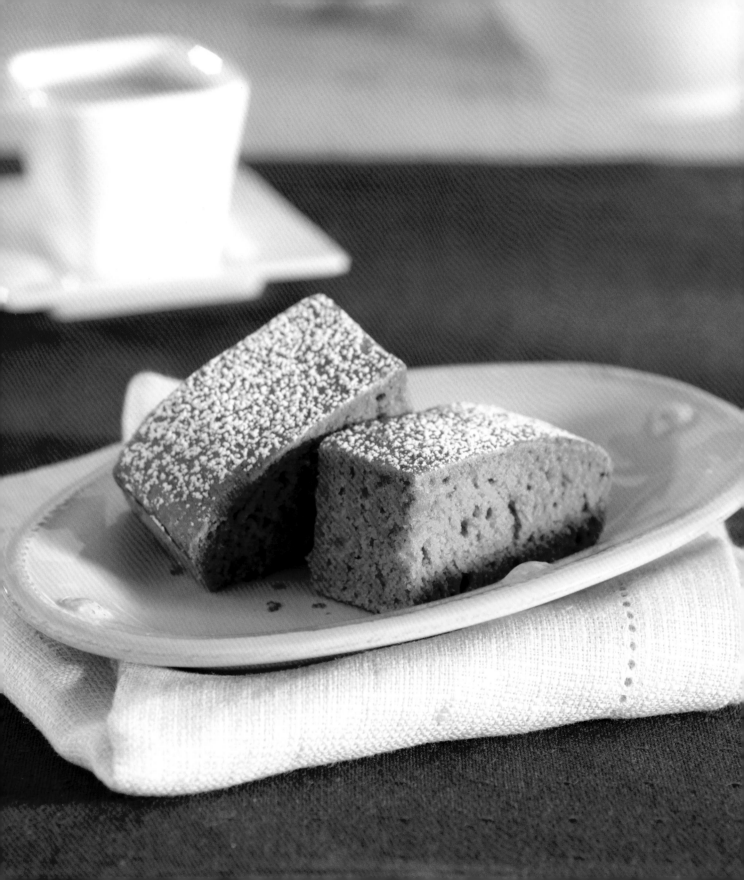

FRUIT FREEZIES

MAKES 12 SERVINGS

---

1 can (15 ounces) apricot halves in light syrup, rinsed and drained

¾ cup apricot nectar

3 tablespoons sugar, divided

Round or square ice cube trays

1 can (15 ounces) sliced pears in light syrup, rinsed and drained

¾ cup pear nectar

1½ cups frozen chopped mango

¾ cup mango nectar

Picks or mini pop sticks

---

1 Combine apricots, apricot nectar and 1 tablespoon sugar in blender or food processor; blend until smooth. Pour mixture evenly into one third of ice cube trays (8 cubes).

2 Combine pears, pear nectar and 1 tablespoon sugar in blender or food processor; blend until smooth. Pour mixture evenly into one third of ice cube trays (8 cubes).

3 Combine mango, mango nectar and remaining 1 tablespoon sugar in blender or food processor; blend until smooth. Pour mixture evenly into remaining one third of ice cube tray (8 cubes).

4 Freeze 1 to 2 hours or until almost firm.

5 Insert picks. Freeze 1 to 2 hours or until firm.

6 To remove pops from trays, place bottoms of ice cube trays under warm running water until loosened. Press firmly on bottoms to release. (Do not twist or pull picks.)

VARIATION: Try any of these favorite fruit combinations or create your own! Use crushed pineapple and pineapple juice or add more flavor to the combinations above. Add coconut extract to the apricot mixture or almond extract to the pear mixture.

NUTRIENTS PER SERVING:

Calories: 19, **Total Fat:** 1g, **Saturated Fat:** 1g, **Cholesterol:** 0mg, **Sodium:** 2mg, **Carbohydrates:** 5g, **Dietary Fiber:** 1g, **Protein:** 1g
Dietary Exchange: ½ Fruit

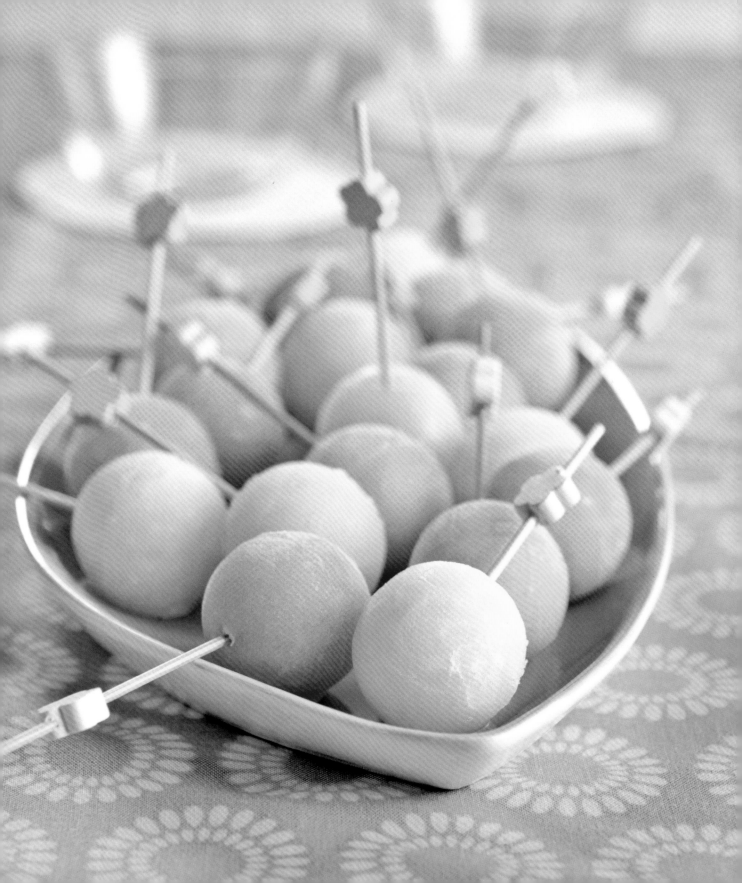

SOUR CREAM APPLE TART

MAKES 12 SERVINGS

- 5 tablespoons light margarine, divided
- ¾ cup graham cracker crumbs
- 1¼ teaspoons ground cinnamon, divided
- 1⅓ cups reduced-fat sour cream
- ¾ cup sugar, divided
- ½ cup all-purpose flour, divided
- ½ cup cholesterol-free egg substitute
- 1 teaspoon vanilla
- 5 cups coarsely chopped peeled Jonathan apples or other firm red-skinned apples

1. Preheat oven to 350°F.

2. Melt 3 tablespoons margarine in small saucepan over medium heat. Stir in graham cracker crumbs and ¼ teaspoon cinnamon until well blended. Press crumb mixture firmly onto bottom of 9-inch springform pan. Bake 10 minutes. Remove to wire rack to cool.

3. Beat sour cream, ½ cup sugar and 2 tablespoons plus 1½ teaspoons flour in large bowl with electric mixer at medium speed until well blended. Beat in egg substitute and vanilla until well blended. Stir in apples. Spoon into prepared crust.

4. Bake 35 minutes or just until center is set. Cut into 12 slices.

5. Preheat broiler. Combine remaining 1 teaspoon cinnamon, ¼ cup sugar and 5 tablespoons plus 1½ teaspoons flour in small bowl. Cut in remaining 2 tablespoons margarine with pastry blender until mixture resembles coarse crumbs. Sprinkle over top of pie.

6. Broil 3 to 4 minutes or until topping is golden brown. Let stand 15 minutes before serving.

NUTRIENTS PER SERVING:

Calories: 180, **Total Fat:** 5g, **Saturated Fat:** 1g, **Cholesterol:** 8mg, **Sodium:** 124mg, **Carbohydrates:** 30g, **Dietary Fiber:** 1g, **Protein:** 3g
Dietary Exchange: 1½ Bread/Starch, ½ Fruit, 1 Fat

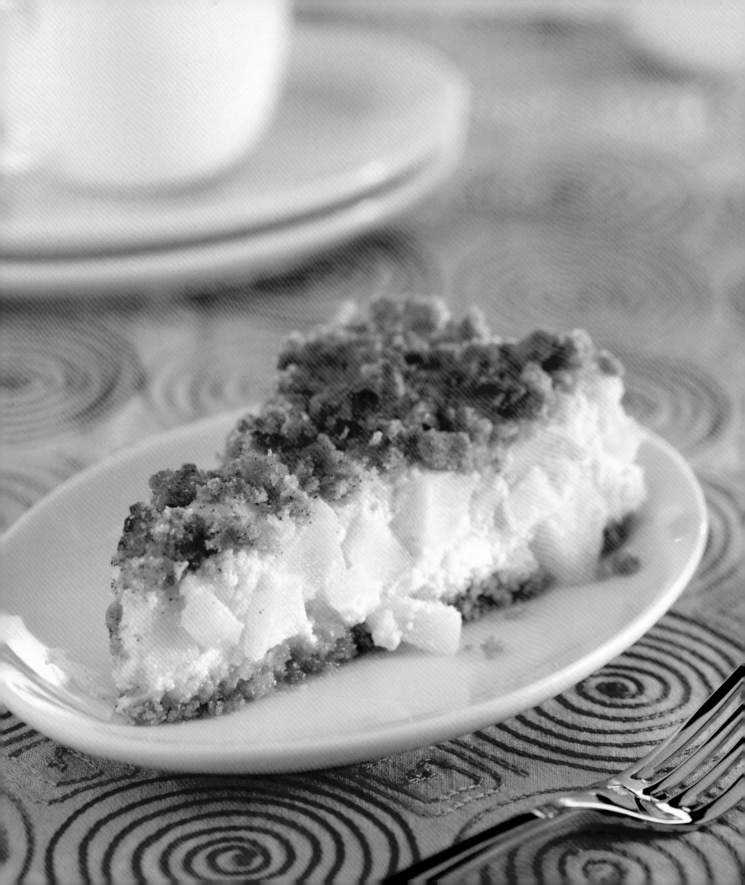

CHOCOLATE ANGEL FRUIT TORTE

MAKES 12 SERVINGS

---

1 package (about 16 ounces) angel food cake mix

½ cup unsweetened cocoa powder

2 bananas, thinly sliced

1½ teaspoons lemon juice

1 can (12 ounces) evaporated skim milk, divided

⅓ cup sugar

¼ cup cornstarch

⅓ cup cholesterol-free egg substitute

3 tablespoons fat-free sour cream

3 teaspoons vanilla

3 large kiwis, peeled and thinly sliced

1 can (11 ounces) mandarin orange segments, rinsed and drained

---

1 Prepare and bake cake mix according to package directions, adding cocoa to dry ingredients. Cool completely. Cut cake in half crosswise to create 2 layers.

2 Combine banana slices and lemon juice in medium bowl; toss to coat.

3 Combine ¼ cup evaporated milk, sugar and cornstarch in small saucepan; whisk until smooth. Whisk in remaining evaporated milk. Bring to a boil over high heat, stirring constantly. Boil 1 minute or until mixture thickens, stirring constantly.

4 Beat ⅓ cup hot milk mixture and egg substitute in small bowl until blended. Slowly add to saucepan over medium-low heat; cook 2 minutes, stirring constantly. Remove from heat; let stand 10 minutes, stirring frequently. Stir in sour cream and vanilla until well blended.

5 Place bottom half of cake on serving plate; spread with half of milk mixture. Top with half of banana slices, kiwi slices and mandarin orange segments. Place remaining half of cake, cut side down, over fruit; top with remaining milk mixture and fruit.

NUTRIENTS PER SERVING:

Calories: 233, **Total Fat:** 1g, **Saturated Fat:** 1g, **Cholesterol:** 1mg, **Sodium:** 306mg, **Carbohydrates:** 52g, **Dietary Fiber:** 1g, **Protein:** 7g
Dietary Exchange: 2½ Bread/Starch, 1 Fruit

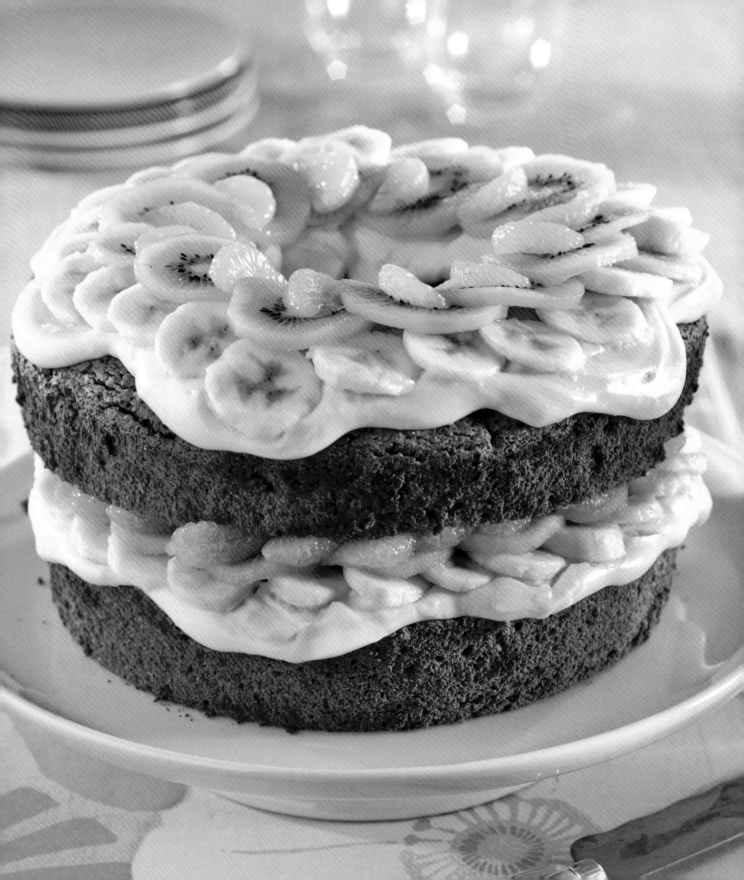

LEMON RASPBERRY TIRAMISÙ

MAKES 12 SERVINGS

2 packages (8 ounces each) fat-free cream cheese, softened

6 packets sugar substitute *or* equivalent of ¼ cup sugar

1 teaspoon vanilla

⅓ cup water

1 package (4-serving size) sugar-free lemon-flavored gelatin

2 cups thawed frozen fat-free nondairy whipped topping

½ cup red raspberry preserves

¼ cup water

2 tablespoons marsala wine

2 packages (3 ounces each) ladyfingers

2 cups fresh raspberries or frozen unsweetened raspberries, thawed, divided

1 Beat cream cheese, sugar substitute and vanilla in large bowl with electric mixer at high speed until smooth.

2 Combine water and gelatin in small microwavable bowl; microwave on HIGH 30 seconds to 1 minute or until water is boiling and gelatin is dissolved. Cool slightly.

3 Add gelatin mixture to cream cheese mixture; beat 1 minute. Add whipped topping; beat 1 minute.

4 Whisk preserves, water and marsala in small bowl until well blended. Reserve 2 tablespoons preserves mixture; set aside. Spread ⅓ cup preserves mixture evenly over bottom of 11×7-inch baking dish.

5 Split ladyfingers in half; arrange half over preserves in baking dish. Spread half of cheese mixture evenly over ladyfingers; sprinkle with 1 cup raspberries. Top with remaining ladyfingers; spread remaining preserves mixture over ladyfingers. Top with remaining cheese mixture. Cover and refrigerate at least 2 hours. Drizzle with reserved 2 tablespoons preserves mixture and sprinkle with remaining raspberries before serving.

NUTRIENTS PER SERVING:

Calories: 158, **Total Fat:** 1g, **Saturated Fat:** 1g, **Cholesterol:** 52mg, **Sodium:** 272mg, **Carbohydrates:** 26g, **Dietary Fiber:** 1g, **Protein:** 7g
Dietary Exchange: 2 Bread/Starch

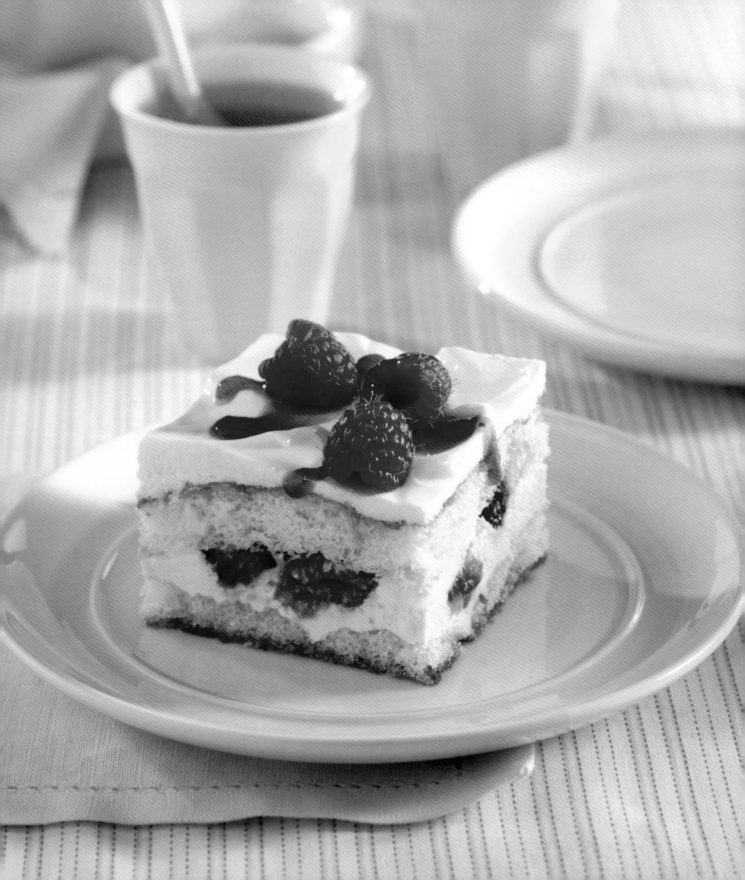

STRAWBERRY CHEESECAKE PARFAITS

MAKES 4 SERVINGS

1½ cups vanilla nonfat Greek yogurt

½ cup whipped cream cheese, at room temperature

2 tablespoons powdered sugar

1 teaspoon vanilla

2 cups sliced fresh strawberries

2 teaspoons granulated sugar

8 honey graham cracker squares, coarsely crumbled (about 2 cups)

Fresh mint leaves (optional)

---

1 Whisk yogurt, cream cheese, powdered sugar and vanilla in small bowl until smooth and well blended.

2 Combine strawberries and granulated sugar in small bowl; gently toss.

3 Layer ¼ cup yogurt mixture, ¼ cup strawberries and ¼ cup graham cracker crumbs in each of 4 dessert dishes. Repeat layers. Garnish with mint. Serve immediately.

NUTRIENTS PER SERVING:

Calories: 220, **Total Fat:** 7g, **Saturated Fat:** 3g, **Cholesterol:** 15mg, **Sodium:** 200mg, **Carbohydrates:** 29g, **Dietary Fiber:** 2g, **Protein:** 11g
Dietary Exchange: 1 Bread/Starch, 1 Fruit, 1 Fat

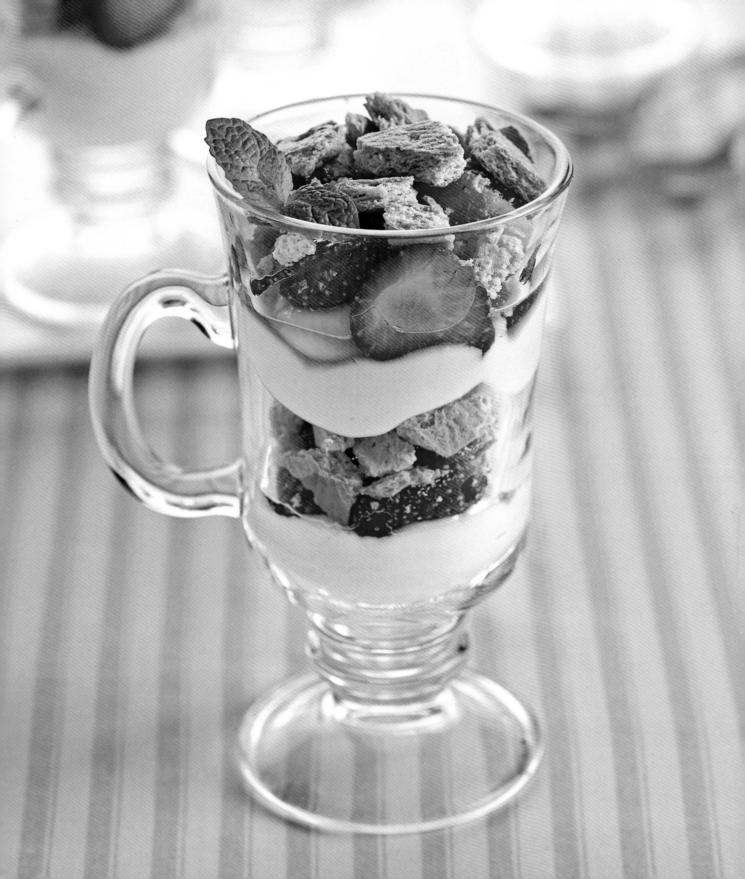

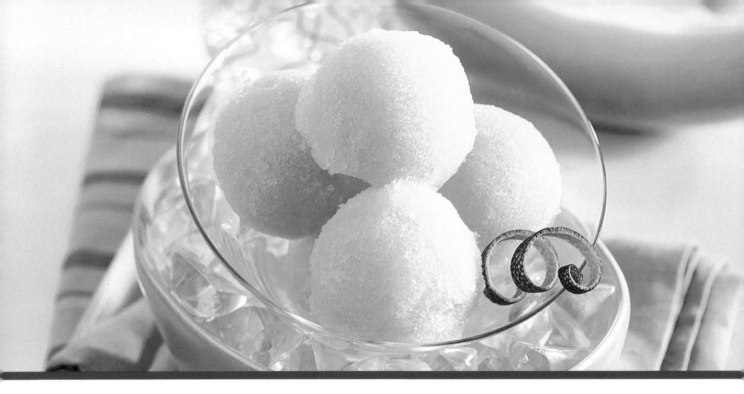

HONEYDEW MELON SORBET

MAKES 8 SERVINGS

⅔ **cup water**

⅔ **cup sugar substitute**

4 **teaspoons lemon juice**

1 **honeydew melon**

1 Combine water, sugar substitute and lemon juice in small saucepan; bring to a boil over medium-high heat. Boil 1 minute. Set aside 15 minutes to cool to room temperature.

2 Remove rind and seeds from melon. Cut melon into pieces. Place melon in food processor or blender; process until smooth. Add sugar substitute mixture; process until combined. Pour into 8-inch square baking pan.

3 Freeze at least 4 hours or overnight. Let stand at room temperature 15 minutes to soften slightly before serving. Scoop into dessert dishes.

NUTRIENTS PER SERVING:

Calories: 46, **Total Fat:** 0g, **Saturated Fat:** 0g, **Cholesterol:** 0mg, **Sodium:** 23mg, **Carbohydrates:** 14g, **Dietary Fiber:** 1g, **Protein:** 1g
Dietary Exchange: 1 Fruit

Index

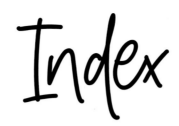

Metric Conversion Chart

VOLUME MEASUREMENTS (dry)

¹⁄₈ teaspoon = 0.5 mL
¹⁄₄ teaspoon = 1 mL
¹⁄₂ teaspoon = 2 mL
³⁄₄ teaspoon = 4 mL
1 teaspoon = 5 mL
1 tablespoon = 15 mL
2 tablespoons = 30 mL
¹⁄₄ cup = 60 mL
¹⁄₃ cup = 75 mL
¹⁄₂ cup = 125 mL
²⁄₃ cup = 150 mL
³⁄₄ cup = 175 mL
1 cup = 250 mL
2 cups = 1 pint = 500 mL
3 cups = 750 mL
4 cups = 1 quart = 1 L

VOLUME MEASUREMENTS (fluid)

1 fluid ounce (2 tablespoons) = 30 mL
4 fluid ounces (¹⁄₂ cup) = 125 mL
8 fluid ounces (1 cup) = 250 mL
12 fluid ounces (1¹⁄₂ cups) = 375 mL
16 fluid ounces (2 cups) = 500 mL

WEIGHTS (mass)

¹⁄₂ ounce = 15 g
1 ounce = 30 g
3 ounces = 90 g
4 ounces = 120 g
8 ounces = 225 g
10 ounces = 285 g
12 ounces = 360 g
16 ounces = 1 pound = 450 g

DIMENSIONS

¹⁄₁₆ inch = 2 mm
¹⁄₈ inch = 3 mm
¹⁄₄ inch = 6 mm
¹⁄₂ inch = 1.5 cm
³⁄₄ inch = 2 cm
1 inch = 2.5 cm

OVEN TEMPERATURES

250°F = 120°C
275°F = 140°C
300°F = 150°C
325°F = 160°C
350°F = 180°C
375°F = 190°C
400°F = 200°C
425°F = 220°C
450°F = 230°C

BAKING PAN SIZES

Utensil	Size in Inches/Quarts	Metric Volume	Size in Centimeters
Baking or Cake Pan (square or rectangular)	8×8×2	2 L	20×20×5
	9×9×2	2.5 L	23×23×5
	12×8×2	3 L	30×20×5
	13×9×2	3.5 L	33×23×5
Loaf Pan	8×4×3	1.5 L	20×10×7
	9×5×3	2 L	23×13×7
Round Layer Cake Pan	8×1½	1.2 L	20×4
	9×1½	1.5 L	23×4
Pie Plate	8×1¼	750 mL	20×3
	9×1¼	1 L	23×3
Baking Dish or Casserole	1 quart	1 L	—
	1½ quart	1.5 L	—
	2 quart	2 L	—